SOCIAL LIFE AND MORAL JUDGMENT

SOCIAL LIFE AND MORAL JUDGMENT

Antony Flew

Routledge
Taylor & Francis Group
LONDON AND NEW YORK

First published 2003 by Transaction Publishers

2 Park Square, Milton Park, Abingdon, Oxfordshire OX14 4RN
711 Third Avenue, New York, NY 10017

Routledge is an imprint of the Taylor & Francis Group, an informa business

First issued in paperback 2017

Library of Congress Catalog Number: 2002075922

Library of Congress Cataloging-in-Publication Data

Flew, Antony, 1923-
Social life and moral judgment / Antony Flew.
p. cm.
Includes bibliographical references and index.
ISBN 0-7658-0155-8 (alk. paper)
1. Public welfare—Philosophy. 2. Public welfare—Moral and ethical aspects. 3. Welfare state—Moral and ethical aspects. 4. Social justice. I. Title.

HV31 .F55 2003
361.6'14—dc21 2002075922

ISBN 13: 978-0-7658-0155-5 (hbk)
ISBN 13: 978-1-138-51471-3 (pbk)

Contents

Introduction and Acknowledgements

Social Life and Moral Judgment is a collection of essays united by their relevance to the problems of mature welfare states. Its purpose is to contribute to struggles against the hypertrophy of these institutions and for their progressive privatization. Its particular contribution is to concentrate upon their demoralizing effects.

Chapter 1 asks "Is Human Sociobiology Possible?" and answers that it is not. For we human beings are all members of a peculiar kind of creatures who can, and therefore cannot but, make and thus become responsible for our individual choices between the various possible courses of action or inaction which are from time to time open to us. Chapters 2, 3, and 4 all show how state welfare systems inevitably demoralize both by encouraging ever more citizens to apply for their welfare "entitlements" and by reducing the incentives to avoid or escape the conditions qualifying them for these "entitlements." Chapter 5, "Welfare Rights for the Formerly Disadvantaged," examines the origins of this new kind of welfare entitlement, a new kind which while making no fresh direct demands upon the taxpayers instead imposes arbitrary and unpredictable burdens upon employers.

Chapter 6, "Sincerity, Rationality, and Monitoring," applies these related ideas to various sets of both politicians and public sector employees to show how very different what these people actually produce is from the goods they pretend to be producing. It could therefore be seen as opening a new sub-branch of the economics of public choice. Chapter 7, "Selfishness, Exploitation, and the Profit Motive," strives to discredit those who labor to discredit wealth creation. The penultimate chapter 8 argues that "social" justice, which apparently requires that everyone's justly acquired income and wealth should be so taxed away or tax-supplemented that the result is ever more though never perfect equality of after-tax income, is a fundamentally different principle from that of old-fashioned, without prefix or suffix, justice. It was justice in that traditional understanding of which Adam Smith famously said that it is a virtue "of which the observance is not left to the freedom of our wills" but "which may be extorted by force." So the moral of the concluding chapter 9, "Moral Education in Secular State Schools," is that the necessary and perhaps sufficient syllabus for moral education in such schools cannot but consist of the principles of that old-fashioned, without prefix or suffix, justice; obedience to which both can and must be presented as obligatory upon everyone everywhere, and not as merely relative to any particular time or place.

What follows is a new book rather than a collection of reprinted papers. It does, nevertheless, contain much material recycled from various publications. Thanks are therefore owed, and gladly given, to all the editors and publishers who have granted their permission for this reuse.

Chapter 1 is a revision of the article "Is Human Sociobiology Possible?" which originally appeared in Volume 25 of *Philosophy of the Social Sciences*, a journal published by Sage Publications of Thousand Oaks, CA. Chapter 2 was developed from "Anti-Social Determinism," which appeared first in 1994 in *Philosophy*, a journal published by the Royal Institute of Philosophy, London. Chapter 3 was developed from "State Welfare and Individual Demoralization," originally published in Volume VI of the *Journal des Economistes et des Etudes Humaines* under the auspices of L'Institut European des Etudes Humaines of Aix en Provence, France. This article was reprinted in Gerard Radnitzky and Hardy Bouillon (eds.) *Values and The Social Order*, Vol. 3, published by Avebury. Avebury is an arm of Ashgate Publishers of Aldershot, England.

Chapter 4 draws on materials from two publications of the Social Affairs Unit, London: *Self-improvement and Social Action*, a pamphlet published in 1989; and "Self-improvement: and its neglect by the contemporary mainstream churches," a chapter in the book *The Loss of Virtue: Moral Confusion and Social Disorder in Britain and America*, published in 1993. Chapter 5 draws on materials both from a Critical Notice of Richard Epstein's *Forbidden Grounds: The Case against Employment Discrimination Laws* in *Reason Papers 1994* (a journal published under the auspices of the *Reason* Foundation of Los Angeles) and from "Animal rights: nonsense on stilts," a chapter in Michael Mosbacher and Digby Anderson (eds.) *Another Country*, a 1999 publication of the Social Affairs Unit.

Chapter 6 starts from an article, "Do-gooders doing no good?" in Catherine Jones and Maria Brenton (eds.) *The Year Book of Social Policy in Britain 1984-5*, published in 1985 by Routledge under their earlier incarnation of Routledge and Kegan Paul. Chapter 7 consists in an extensively revised version of an article under the same title that was originally included in a collection of essays on *Business Ethics and Common Sense*, edited by Robert McGee and published in 1992 by Quorum Books, an arm of the Greenwood Publishing Group of Westport, CT. Chapter 8 is a radically revised version of an article on "Private Property and 'Social' Justice" included in a collection of essays entitled *The Idea of Property in History and Modern Times*. This collection was edited by His Honour Colin Kolbert and published by the Ian Mactaggart Trust in Glasgow and the Churchill Press in London. Finally, chapter 9 has not been previously published.

1

Is Human Sociobiology Possible?

Sociobiology is defined as the systematic study of the biological basis of all social behavior.—E. O. Wilson, Sociobiology: The New Synthesis *(p. 4)*

The second word in the title of this first chapter is crucial. For there can be no doubt but that the possibility of sociobiology below the human level has already been abundantly realized in, for instance, the main body of E. O. Wilson's enormous and encyclopaedic treatise *Sociobiology: The New Synthesis.* What may more reasonably be doubted, and what is about to be questioned here is whether, as Wilson and others hoped and expected, there is much, or indeed any room for a sociobiology of our own notoriously wayward and idiosyncratic species. In proposing and pursuing that project, Wilson and his associates have seen themselves as promoting a climactic conquest for evolutionary biology. For surely, they seem to have thought, it is now, more than a century after Darwin, high time and over time to launch the final assault upon the last citadel.

There are however, as we shall proceed to argue, reasons—reasons which were available at least in outline even to Darwin himself—why the ideas that have been so triumphantly successful in explaining *The Origin of Species* cannot properly be applied to what is in truth a fundamentally different task. They cannot, that is to say, properly be transferred to explain developments either within or out of the particular problem species of which the author of that book, along with both all the authors and all the readers of all other books, have been themselves members. For there are fundamental differences between the natural and the human sciences, the latter including the (human) social sciences. These fundamental differences are consequences of the essential peculiarities of that peculiar species of which we are all members: *homo sapiens*. It is the main purpose of this present chapter and of its immediate successor to elucidate the nature of these peculiarities and their implications for both the understanding and the application of the findings of the (human) social sciences—hereafter described as usually they are, as without qualification, the social sciences.

The Project of Human Sociobiology

By itself, the claim that biology provides the basis of all social behavior might imply everything or almost nothing. The foundations of a building, the basis without which that building must inevitably collapse, place only the broadest and most generous limitations upon what can be erected upon and supported by those foundations. It is also only when archaeologists possess considerable knowledge of the people who built what used to rest upon some still surviving foundations can they begin to make reasonable conjectures about the architecture, the materials, and the function of a structure that exists no longer. At the other extreme, we sometimes used to hear brashly dogmatic Marxists maintaining that the material foundations of any society—its forms of "production and reproduction in real life"—must more or less rigorously determine and necessitate whatever is going on in the ideological superstructure of that society.

In applying sociobiological ideas to the study of human social behavior, Wilson himself, whose own main previous research was on *The Insect Societies*, inclined to the latter extreme. In a final chapter of that earlier book, a chapter surveying the prospects for "a unified sociobiology," he envisaged that "the same principles of population biology and comparative zoology" that had "worked so well in explaining the rigid systems of the social insects could be applied point by point to vertebrate animals."[1] How this application was to be achieved Wilson indicated in the paragraph of *Sociobiology: The New Synthesis* that contained the definition already quoted. It would, apparently, involve a take-over by evolutionary genetics. For "Sociology *sensu stricto*...still stands apart from sociobiology because of its largely...nongenetic approach... Taxonomy and ecology...have been reshaped entirely...by integration into neo-Darwinist evolutionary theory—the 'Modern Synthesis' as it is often called—*in which each phenomenon is weighed for its adaptive significance and then related to the basic principles of population genetics.*"[2] This particular paragraph, however, concluded cautiously: "Whether the social sciences can be truly biologicized in this fashion remains to be seen."

In subsequent writings Wilson was less cautious and more explicit in his reductionist ambitions. Biology, he later went on to argue, is the "antidiscipline" of the social sciences, and of anthropology in particular, "which has already become the social science closest to sociobiology."[3] It is, it seems, the scientific function of an antidiscipline to reduce to its own level the explanations of the science next above it. So it falls to sociobiology, as the antidiscipline of anthropology, to demonstrate that the explanation of cultural practices is really to be found in biological processes. The issue at stake is the extent to which human cultures, and the behaviors that are elements in them, can be accounted for by "genetic determinism." It is on the interpretation of this "key phrase," as Wilson stressed, that "the entire relation between biology and the social sciences depends" (E. O. Wilson, 1978, p. 55).

The final chapter of *Sociobiology: The New Synthesis* is entitled "Man: From Sociobiology to Sociology." It gets off to a splendid start with the sentence: "Let us now consider man in the free spirit of natural history, as though we were zoologists from another planet completing a catalog of social species on Earth" (E. O. Wilson, 1975, p. 547). Unfortunately, after having so rightly and so immediately insisted that this is what needed to be done, Wilson did not, either then or later, go on to actually do it. Instead, he proceeded by his subsequent off-the-cuff remarks about human nature to provoke explosions of fury from various individuals and collectives committed to the defense of social democratic or Marxist orthodoxies. No doubt Wilson himself saw this reaction as clear confirmation for his claim that human beings are "absurdly easy to indoctrinate."[4]

How to Inherit Acquired Characteristics

What needed to be done but was not done, either by Wilson himself or even by Kitcher[5]—by far the most well-girded and fair-minded of all Wilson's critics—was to ask which, if any, of the distinctive peculiarities of our species are or should be of especial professional interest to biologists. Suppose now that we actually were to begin, as Wilson, on the first page of the final chapter of *Sociobiology: The New Synthesis*, recommended that we should begin, by considering "man in the free spirit of natural history, as though we were zoologists from another planet completing a catalog of social species on Earth." Then the first peculiarities we would have to pick out would surely be the far-extended period between birth and maturity, the incomparable capacity for learning that makes it possible to take full advantage of that far-extended period, and the consequent importance of learned (as opposed to instinctual) behavior. Our unrivalled capacity for learning, together with its instrument and expression developed language, provides our species with a serviceable substitute for the (genetic) inheritance of acquired characteristics.

This is a point that seems first to have been made, very forcefully, by Julian Huxley.[6] His making it in 1923 is all the more impressive in that he was at that time much concerned to put down all Lamarckist suggestions that any acquired characteristics might be (genetically) inherited. It is this serviceable substitute for the (genetic) inheritance of acquired characteristics that constitutes the first threat to the project for a human sociobiology. For the genetic inheritance of acquired characteristics itself, as opposed to this or any other substitute, is something most emphatically precluded by—Huxley's phrase—the "Modern Synthesis."

No doubt this unrivalled capacity for learning, like all other innate capacities and innate dispositions, is itself genetically determined. But the directions to which *we* turn such capacities, and how far *we* inhibit or pursue such inclinations, is precisely not already determined by our genes. It is instead for us to decide. And in this, as we shall see in the following section, lies the second main threat to the project for a human sociobiology.

It is perhaps significant that Wilson here mentions only sociology and anthropology as the disciplines or discipline for which sociobiology is to be the antidiscipline. For different reasons, neither of these makes much room for history or tradition. Yet fully to understand any human as opposed to insect society it is essential to take account of its past. In the oft-quoted words with which Marx begins the second paragraph of *The Eighteenth Brumaire of Louis Bonaparte*:

> Men make their own history, but they do not make it just as they please; they do not make it under circumstances chosen by themselves, but under circumstances directly encountered, given and transmitted from the past. The tradition of all the dead generations weighs like a nightmare[7] on the brain of the living (Marx [1852] 1934, p. 10).

What is peculiar to our species, it must be emphasized, is not the exogenetic (i.e. non-genetic) transmission of specific possible behaviors from one generation to the next, as such, but the enormous number and variety of possible behaviors which, thanks to the hypertrophy of the human brain and to the presumably concurrent and connected development of language, can now be and often are transmitted exogenetically. Wilson himself is, of course, far too good a biologist not to have noticed both what is and what is not peculiar to our species. What he noticed in *Sociobiology: The New Synthesis* is that populations of primates and other animals possess traditions, "specific forms of behavior that are passed from generation to generation by learning," by processes, that is, which are specifically exogenetic. These traditions, when viewed collectively, constitute the culture of an animal population; and, as Wilson also notices, from the researches of primatologists during recent decades, it has now been established that "the rudiments of culture are possessed by higher primates other than man, including the Japanese monkey and the chimpanzee" (E. O. Wilson, 1975, p. 168).

For populations of both the Japanese monkey and the chimpanzee, we now possess decisive evidence of the exogenetic transmission of information between successive generations.[8] Moreover, the fact that the information transmitted is rudimentary in form is of particular significance when seen in an evolutionary perspective. For in both of these meticulously documented cases we are given a glimpse of the way in which the cultural transmission of information emerges: through the operation of entirely natural processes from pre-existing genetically determined adaptations. The fact that Wilson himself noticed the emergence of this phenomenon of exogenetic cultural inheritance at an infrahuman level made it all the more remarkable, not to say mildly scandalous, that he should then seem not to see the significance for his own ambitious project of the explosive, exponential growth of the same phenomenon at human level.

How to Frustrate Your Genes

Many and various are the differentials that have been suggested in order to produce *per genus et differentiam* definitions expressing what the definers took to be an, if not *the*, essential peculiarity of our species. Such differentials have usually been chosen in order to maintain the purportedly objective centrality of whatever happened to be the chief interest of the chooser. Thus we have been categorized under the class-descriptions of "the religious animal," "the animal which knows it has to die," and innumerable others. Quite the best for our present purpose is the first. It was, appropriately enough, the one provided by the Founding Father of biological science.

For Aristotle proposed to define and distinguish man as "the rational animal." Here the word "rational" has to be construed as meaning capable of rationality, and it is opposed (not to the word "irrational" but) to the word "non-rational." For us, the prime implication of this definition is that man becomes essentially a language-using creature. But Aristotle also distinguished two sorts of reason: theoretical and practical. Both of these are equally essential to man, and both of course presuppose linguistic capacities. Practical reason is reason in and for action: it is a matter of the reasons one may have for acting or not acting, or for acting in this way rather than that. To possess and to be able to employ practical reason presupposes that one is an *agent*, rather than a mere patient. But to act—as opposed to merely behaving in the way in which, we presume, the brutes merely behave—is always and necessarily to be able to do otherwise than in fact we do do. Creatures which are, in this understanding, agents are, therefore, a kind of creatures which can, and cannot but, make choices; and which may have and know that they have practical reasons for making the particular choices they do make in the senses in which they do make them. It is thus certain fundamental defining and distinguishing peculiarities of our species, rather than the offensiveness of its findings to various militant ideologies, which must necessarily frustrate all aspirations to develop a human sociobiology.

The first biologically relevant peculiarity of our species here distinguished is our capacity to inherit some acquired characteristics. The second biologically relevant peculiarity of our species is that we are all, to a greater or lesser extent, agents. Since agents as such always could—in a strong sense that will be explained in chapter 2—have done and could do other than they did do and do do, there sometimes arise for all of us possibilities of, as it were, frustrating our genes. Presumably there are in some non-human mammals embryonic developments in this direction—just as, as we have seen, there certainly are cases of the exogenetic inheritance of the acquired characteristic of a learned behavior in several species other than ours. In both instances, however, the prehuman anticipations of what has in our species become a vastly extended and elaborately sophisticated development appear to be comparatively minor. It is this second peculiarity of our species, even more than the first, which makes the human sciences irreducibly different from the natural. In his own way, Wilson recognized the reality of choice. But, once again, he failed altogether to appreciate its revolutionary and relevant significance.

As was said before, the issue at stake is the extent to which human cultures, and the behaviors that are part of them, can be explained in terms of "genetic determinism." It is on the interpretation of this "key phrase," as Wilson stressed, that the entire relation between biology and social sciences depends (E. O. Wilson, 1975, p. 532). As an example of an organism whose behavior is genetically "predestined," he instanced the mosquito: "The mosquito," he wrote, "is an automaton" with "a sequence of rigid behaviors programmed by the genes to unfold swiftly and unerringly from birth to the final act of oviposition" (E. O. Wilson, 1987, p. 55).

He then immediately went on to take as an example of "restricted behavior" in humans the phenomenon of handedness: "Each person is biologically predisposed to be either left or right handed" (E. O. Wilson, 1978, p. 57). Nevertheless, as he himself notes, while parents in present-day Western societies tend not to interfere with the "direction set by the gene affecting this trait," the position is decidedly different in "traditional Chinese societies," in which "a strong social pressure for right-handed writing and eating" is still exerted. Thus, a then-recent study of Taiwanese children[9] "found a nearly complete conformity in these two activities, but little or no effect on handedness in other activities not subjected to special training" (E. O. Wilson, 1978, p. 57).

The conclusion Wilson drew from this instructive example is that, in the case of the "restricted behavior" of handedness, "the genes have their way unless specifically contravened by conscious choice" (E. O. Wilson, 1978, p. 57). But it will not do, as he did, to leave it at that. For whenever genes have causally necessitated their, shall we say, owners, or subjects, or whatever else, to have not uncontrollable reflexes, but inhibitable and controllable desires or dispositions or orientations or inclinations, then this must open the possibility that choice will intervene to contravene. So there is now no longer any necessitarian determination of the consequent behavior.

The first essential here is to distinguish two crucially different senses of the word "cause," and then, after that, two correspondingly different senses of the word "determinism." For there is an absolutely fundamental difference: between, on the one hand, ensuring that some person will act in one particular way, by providing them with some overwhelmingly strong practical reason so to do; and, on the other hand, making some purely physical phenomenon happen, by bringing about the causally sufficient conditions of its occurrence. Let us, following Hume's suggestion in his essay "Of National Characters," distinguish these two kinds of cause as moral and physical: "By *moral* causes, I mean all circumstances, which are fitted to work on the mind as motives or reasons... By *physical* causes I mean those qualities of the air and climate, which are supposed to work insensibly on the temper, by altering the tone and habit of the body..." (Hume [1742-77], 1985, p. 198: emphases original).

The absolutely fundamental difference between these two kinds is that, whereas sufficient physical causes necessarily necessitate the occurrence of their effects, correspondingly sufficient moral causes do not. If, for instance, I convey to you some splendid news—news the reception of which, if you decided to celebrate, you and everyone else would point to as the cause of that celebration—then I do not by so doing ensure that you must, whether or not you want to, celebrate. Actions that are thus caused by moral causes are neither uncaused nor necessarily capricious and inexplicable, although, inasmuch as they are indeed actions, it is impossible for them to be physically necessitated. It is equally mistaken to assume—as most professing social scientists, apparently, do assume—that all environmental causes are, in the sense explained, physical and therefore physically necessitating, and therefore, because physically necessitating, excusing.

Corresponding to these two radically different senses of the word "cause" are two similarly different understandings of the term "determinism": what is determined by physical causes *must*, whereas what is determined by moral causes *cannot*, be physically necessitated. These two distinctions are essential for any adequate understanding of the fundamental and irreducible differences between the natural and the human sciences; and for an appreciation of what is and is not implied by any discoveries that professors of the latter may claim to have made about the causes of marriage breakdown, war, juvenile or adult delinquency, or any of the other myriad ills to which the flesh is heir. If, having their reasons for acting, people act—whether creditably or discreditably, or neither—then it cannot have been physically impossible for them to have done other than they did. If this was not true of their behaviors, then those behaviors cannot have constituted instances of human action.

It is extremely important to get and to keep a firm hold upon the three ideas of agency, choice, and physical necessity. For the first two, which are both essential to and central in the human sciences, are both incompatible with the third, which is equally essential to and central in the natural sciences. So by further elucidating these and other related concepts in chapter 2 we shall not only be reinforcing the contention that the project for a human sociobiology must be aborted but also developing the implications of the contention that the human sciences cannot be reduced to the natural.

Two Kinds of Power

Anyone wondering what these philosophical distinguishings have to do with biology in general and sociobiology in particular may be reminded of the fact that both Darwin and Wallace recorded that it was their reading of Malthus that provided the directive stimulus to their theory construction. Much of the compelling force of *An Essay on the Principle of Population* depended upon the failure to distinguish two senses of the word "power."

In one sense, the sense in which the word can be applied to inanimate objects and to most of animate nature, a power simply is a disposition to behave in such-and-such a way, given that such and such conditions are satisfied. Thus we might say that the bomb ("the nuclear device") dropped at Nagasaki possessed an explosive power equivalent to so many tons of TNT, or that a full weight nylon climbing rope has a breaking strain of (a power to hold up to) 4500 pounds. Let us, for future ready reference, label this "power (physical)." In another sense, the sense in which the word is typically applied to people, and perhaps to people only, a power is an ability at will to do or to abstain from doing whatever it may be. Let this be "power (personal)."

What stimulated Darwin to develop his theory of evolution by natural selection was his reading of a famous essay by Thomas Malthus. But right from the start Darwin recognized the crucial difference between the multiplicative power of human and of non-human populations. In terms of the distinction just developed, the former are powers (personal) whereas the latter are powers physical. Much of the compelling force of *An Essay on the Principle of Population*, now usually described as the *First Essay*,[10] derives from its treating this principle of population in man as if it were a power (physical). Later Malthus corrected this mistake by introducing his peculiarly restricted notion of moral restraint into the greatly revised and expanded version of 1802—now usually distinguished as the *Second Essay*. By contrast, Darwin seized upon both the difference and its importance for distinguishing men from the brutes immediately and without hesitation. Thus, in *The Origin of Species*, he argues that "A struggle for existence inevitably follows from the high rate at which all organic beings tend to increase...there must in every case be a struggle for existence..." This is "the doctrine of Malthus applied with manifold force to the whole animal and vegetable kingdoms; *for in this case there can be no artificial increase of food and no prudential restraint from marriage*" (Darwin, [1959] 1968, pp. 116-7: emphasis added).

Already even when he was only just beginning to elaborate his own theory, Darwin grasped both the importance and some of the relevant implications of the facts that persons are possessed of powers (personal), that we, and presumably we alone, can choose consciously and for reasons; we can—that is to say—in the full and unqualified sense select. Darwin's natural selection is no more selection, in this original understanding, than Adam Smith's invisible hand is the hand of Invisible Providence. Both conceptions were, of course, introduced in order to explain how what might look as if it must have resulted from intelligent design could, and perhaps could not but, have been produced without the exercise of any such peculiarly human or super human powers.

It is also worth saying here: both that evolutionary as opposed to creationist ideas were triumphantly applied in the area first of the social rather than the biological sciences, and that Darwin himself appears to have been not only acquainted with but also influenced by some of these successful applications. It was, for instance, in 1787 that Sir William Jones published his discovery of the common descent of the Indo-European languages, and by the time that this had, in 1816, been elaborated by Franz Bopp, the concept of cultural evolution had become a commonplace.[11]

Through the exercise of those vastly superior capacities for learning that our genes have given us, and thanks to the exploitation of the privileged possibilities for the exogenetic inheritance of what has been learned, the extent of the powers in human hands, and the consequent scope of actual and unavoidable choices, have, since Darwin's day, vastly increased. In his day, for instance, the impact both of environmentally destructive human activities and of (what has now to be qualified as artificially) selective breeding was comparatively limited, whereas it has since become ruefully true that our species "has certainly won the contest between animal species in that it is only on [human] sufferance that any other species exist at all, among species large enough to be seen at any rate" (Quinton, in Ramsey 1966, p. 120).

After many long years of seeking in evolutionary biology some secular substitute for a God—for as Matthew Arnold put it, "something not ourselves which makes for righteousness"—Julian Huxley eventually, towards the end of his life, reached a very different and more realistic conclusion: "In the light of evolutionary biology man can now see himself as the sole agent for further evolutionary advance on this planet... He finds himself in the unexpected position of business manager for the cosmic process of evolution" (Huxley, 1953, p. 132). Yet even this statement remains far too weak for an agnostic such as Huxley. For it still suggests that there is a pre-existent scheme of things, that unalterable objectives have been previously set for an enterprise that we just have to manage in a way which ensures that those pre-established and unalterable objectives are achieved. Rather, the truth would appear to be in the concluding words of one of the great sets of Gifford Lectures, that "We have, because human, an inalienable prerogative of responsibility which we cannot devolve, no, not as once was thought, even upon the stars. We can share it only with each other" (Sherrington, [1942] 1951, p. 294).

Notes

1. Wilson, E. O., 1971, pp. 458-60. Here we must not fail to recommend Tullock 1994, a fascinating study of *The Economics of Non-Human Societies* by the co-developer, with James Buchanan, of public choice economics.
2. Wilson, E. O., 1975, p. 4 (emphasis added).
3. Wilson, E. O., "On Biology and the Social Sciences," in *Daedalus* for 1977, pp. 127-40.

4. Wilson, E. O., 1975, p. 562. For a tolerably impartial and detached overview of this whole ferocious controversy, see Montagu 1980.
5. See his 1985 *Vaulting Ambition: Sociobiology and the Quest for Human Nature*.
6. See "Biology and Sociology" in Huxley 1923. In this Huxley said: "By means of tradition-inheritance man is virtually enabled to inherit acquired characters; thus the environment in which the later stages of his development are passed through, and consequently his adult self, the end-product of that development, can be altered far more rapidly than in any other organism."
7. Marx, of course, saw himself as speaking for a revolutionary class. But someone speaking affectionately of the history, institutions, and culture of their own nation would not here employ so dyslogistic a term as "nightmare." It was thus no accident that a man so hostile to any unmodern millennial or other celebration of the institutions and historic achievements of the British people should have become the first prime minister of the United Kingdom to find it necessary to protest his patriotism.
8. See both Itani, J. and Nakamura, A. "The Study of Infrahuman Culture in Japan," in the 1973 Symposia of the 4th International Congress on Primatology, Vol. 1: *Precultural Primate Behavior* and van Lerwick-Goodall, J. "Cultural Elements in a Chimpanzee Community," also in the 1973 Symposia of the 4th International Congress on Primatology, Vol. 1: *Precultural Primate Behavior*.
9. Teng, E. L., Yang, K., and Chang, P. C. "Handedness in Chinese Populations: Biological Social and Pathological Factors," in *Science* for 1976, pp. 1146-50.
10. See, for a full discussion, the Introduction to Malthus [1798] 1970.
11. For Darwin's acquaintance with the work of the Scottish founding fathers of social science, see Flew 1997, pp. 83-92.

2

Anti-Social Determinism

One may deter a criminal by increasing the costs or reducing the benefits of crime, but that strategy does not deal with the "causes" of criminality, and hence does not go to the "root" of the problem. Stated another way, if causal theories explain why a criminal acts as he does, they also explain why he must *act as he does, and therefore they make any reliance on deterrence seem futile or irrelevant.— James Q. Wilson,* Thinking about Crime *(p. 58: emphasis original)*

The general moral decline widely perceived[1] to have been in progress for many years in both the UK and the USA has no doubt, like almost all interesting social phenomena, been an effect of many contributory causes. This chapter attends to only one: the de-moralization more or less unintentionally encouraged by the working of the machinery of the welfare state and then further encouraged by a deliberate and systematic drive to de-moralize both that machinery and what, at least in the UK, its operators have been increasingly inclined to describe as their clients.

Since the 1996 transfer of welfare responsibilities from Washington to the states, extensive and exciting efforts have begun to be made in the USA to check this particular contributing cause of de-moralization; while even in the UK the recently re-elected Prime Minister was, at the time of writing, threatening to introduce triennial tests to determine whether those receiving disability benefits have actually remained unable to work. But none of this removes the need to clarify here and now the conceptual confusions involved in such de-moralization.

What Anti-Social Determinism Is

Suppose we start with Murray's Law of Unintended Rewards. This, as originally formulated, reads: "Any social transfer increases the net value of being in the condition that prompted the transfer" (Charles

Murray, 1984, p. 212). Like the other established laws of economic analysis, this constitutes a logically necessary truth. For as Murray goes on to observe, if "a deficiency is observed—too little money, too little food, too little academic achievement—and a social transfer program tries to fill the gap—with a welfare payment, Food Stamps, a compensating education program," then "the program, however unintentionally, *must* be constructed in such a way that it increases the net value of being in the condition that it seeks to change—either by increasing the rewards or by reducing the penalties" (Ibid., pp. 212-3, emphasis original).

Where the condition prompting some particular program is one to which the patients of that condition could not by their own efforts avoid becoming and/or remaining subject, there is of course no call to take account of Murray's Law of Unintended Rewards. Indeed, the whole point of providing welfare services for, for instance, the blind precisely is to reduce as much as can be the monstrous disvalue of being in a condition into which no one would willingly fall and which, if that were possible, all its victims would strive to escape.

But many of the conditions unintentionally "rewarded" by existing state welfare provisions are conditions into which at least some of their victims could and perhaps ought to have avoided falling and/or which they could and perhaps ought to escape partly or wholly by their own efforts. In so far as this is the case, such rewards must necessarily tend to weaken both any existing inhibitions against falling into these conditions and any existing incentives to escape them. In the case of many of these conditions this alone should be a sufficient cause for concern to maintain and, as far as possible, to strengthen such inhibitions and such incentives.

But for many of those working the machinery of the British welfare state, the supreme commandment seems to have become "Thou shalt not be judgmental."[2] Among such people it appears to be in the highest degree politically incorrect even to suggest the possibility of distinguishing the deserving from the undeserving poor. All welfare payments and services are to be considered as being owed as of right, such rights apparently imposing no reciprocal duties upon the beneficiaries of these payments and services. It has, therefore, been reckoned to be scandalous if there was ever less than a 100 percent uptake by those thus entitled to benefit. It is a perceived scandal that activists both inside and outside that machinery have constantly labored to diminish. Substantial funds have been spent on promoting awareness of individuals' rights to welfare benefits. In theory this is supposed to help the needy who may be ignorant of the assistance available to them, but in practice it creates a climate of opinion in which individuals are encouraged to seek out what they can get and to behave in a way that will justify receiving benefits.

A main support for this systematic and apparently principled demoralization is the assumption of what I want to call "anti-social determinism"; the assumption, that is to say, that the explanations produced by the social and psychological sciences necessarily constitute, at one and the same time, completely sufficient excuses for all the behavior so explained. This is nowadays a very widespread assumption, albeit one which no one is in fact willing and able consistently to maintain, especially, and most significantly, with regard to their political opponents. They are regularly seen as guilty, and without excuse.

People trained in any of those sciences, as many of the operatives of the welfare state machinery have been trained, are apt to feel that this assumption is both required of and justified by their professional qualifications. Perhaps more surprisingly, a spokesman for the Church of England Board for Social Responsibility was, as early as 1975, assuring us that:

> ...concern for man must logically entail a concern for his social condition, and therefore with the social structures and economic organisation of society which are determinants of how people think and behave, and of what happens to them. The sociological insights of Marx, and latterly of B. F. Skinner, should have educated us on this point.[3]

Let us, on this occasion and at this late date, ignore the putative sociological insights of Marx. Presumably the insights of B. F. Skinner are the conclusions or, strictly, the presuppositions of a book with the apt but sinister title *Beyond Freedom and Dignity*.[4] In it, Skinner rejects "the traditional view" that "a person...is autonomous" and "can therefore be held responsible for what he does, and justly punished if he offends." Instead, "A scientific analysis shifts both the responsibility and the achievement to the environment" (Skinner, [1971] 1972, p. 25).

Two Kinds both of Cause and of Determinism

The first need here is to make again, and to develop more fully, two distinctions made earlier. The first was Hume's distinction between moral and physical causes. When we are talking about the causes of some altogether non-human event—say an eclipse of the sun—then we employ the word "cause" in a sense implying both physical necessity and physical impossibility: what happened was physically necessary and anything else was, in the circumstances, physically impossible.

Yet this is precisely not the case with the other sense of "cause": the sense in which we speak of the causes (or reasons or motives) for human actions. Suppose that in bringing welcome news my action is what my hearers, if they choose to respond by celebrating, will quite properly describe as the cause of their celebration. Then I do not by that action of mine make their celebration necessary and their abstention therefrom impossible. To adapt a famous phrase of the philosopher mathematician Gottfried Leibniz, causes of this second, motivating sort incline but do not necessitate. Since Hume denied the legitimacy of the concept of physical necessity, he himself was unable to make this distinction in exactly the same way as it has been made here. Nevertheless, his choice of labels did point towards the fundamental difference between, on the one hand, the natural sciences and, on the other hand, the social and psychological or—as he and his contemporaries would have said—the moral.

Given these two fundamentally different senses of the word "cause," it becomes clear that, at least while we are discussing the behavior of human beings, we now need to distinguish two correspondingly different senses of "determinism": determination by physical causes, and determination by moral causes. Certainly if a piece of behavior (what behaviorists call a behavior) is fully determined by physical causes, then the behaver did not choose to behave in that way. Nor could he, at least at the time when that behavior occurred, have prevented it from occurring. But determination by moral causes is quite another matter. For to explain someone's conduct by reference to their reasons for—that is to say the moral causes of—their acting as they did is to presuppose that they could have acted differently. Desires and wants are certainly not as such irresistible compulsions. Most of us are sufficiently disciplined sometimes to refrain from doing things that we should very much like to do.

It is surely by failing to make these fundamental and crucial distinctions that so many people are misled into construing all explanations of conduct in terms of any kind of cause as tending to support an all-excusing doctrine of universal physical necessitation. If such an anti-social determinism were indeed true, then to understand all would indeed be properly to excuse all. For it would mean that it was physically impossible for anyone to have behaved in any way other than that in which they did behave. And this would constitute an entirely adequate excuse for their behaving in whatever way they actually did behave. But the most commonly suggested social causes of, for instance, (a rise in) crime—poverty, unemployment, boredom, social inequality, lack of educational opportunity, and so on—are all moral causes and hence, to put it exactly as Hume himself put it, "circumstances...fitted to work on the mind as motives or reasons." As such they may well constitute extenuating circumstances. But they certainly cannot necessarily and entirely extinguish individual responsibility.

The second need here is to master the mutually incompatible meanings of both of two massively misleading expressions: "they had no choice," and "they could not have done otherwise." The crux is that the idiomatic application of these expressions is to cases where it is not to be denied, but taken for granted, that, in a profounder sense these agents did have a choice, and could have done otherwise.

"Here I stand. I can no other. So help me God." These most famous words of the archetypal Protestant hero are not to be interpreted (as the French would say if only they spoke English) at the foot of the letter. For Luther was not claiming to have fallen victim to a sudden paralysis—God help him. To say, in the everyday sense of "could not have done otherwise," that I could not have done otherwise, is not merely not inconsistent with but actually presupposes the truth of the assumption that, in a more fundamental sense, I could. What, as really we all know, Luther meant—and indeed said—was: not that he was afflicted with a general paralysis, and hence unable to withdraw, but that none of the alternative courses of action open to him were, to him, acceptable.

Again, consider people who, unlike Luther before the Diet of Worms, act not of their own free will but under some kind and amount of external compulsion or constraint. Take, to reemploy a favourite fictional example, the case of the man who receives from the Godfather "an offer that he cannot refuse." Unlike the errant Mafioso who is without warning gunned down from behind and in that moment ceases to act and to choose, the victimized businessman does have a choice. Is it to be his signature or his brains on the deed to transfer his property to "The Organisation?" Yet, because the alternative rejected was even more intolerable than that accepted, we say that those victims who did put their signatures where the Godfather insisted that they should be put had no choice, that they could not have done otherwise than they did do.

Agency and the Two Kinds of Bodily Movement

So far so good. It should by now have become clear that the reality of choice and the consequent permanent possibility of alternative courses of action, however unacceptable these actual alternatives may sometimes be to the agents concerned, is not threatened by any determination by moral causes. The problems generated by physical causation are more formidable.

The first step is to elucidate the three intimately associated notions of being an agent, having a choice, and being able to do otherwise than in the event that agent actually does do. Perhaps the most promising approach lies by way of the great chapter "Of Power" in Locke's *Essay Concerning Human Understanding*. After by this means completing the elucidation of those three intimately associated notions we shall proceed to distinguish two senses of the word "power": one which makes power an attribute peculiar to people, and the other in which power is manifested only by entities incapable of consciousness or intention. We shall then go on to show that we all of us have the most direct and the most inexpugnably certain personal experience both of physical (as opposed to logical) necessity and of physical (as opposed to logical) impossibility.

Consider the following two passages:

> This at least I think evident, that we find in ourselves a *Power* to begin or forbear, continue or end several...motions of our Bodies... This Power...to prefer the motion of any part of the body to its rest, and *vice versa* in any particular instance, is that which we call the Will (Locke [1690] 1975, II [xxi] 5, p. 236).

> Everyone, I think, finds in himself a *Power* to begin or forebear, continue or put an end to several actions in himself. From the considerations of the extent of this power of the mind over the actions of the Man, which everyone finds in himself, arise the *Ideas of Liberty and Necessity* (Locke [1690] 1975, II [xxi] 5, p. 236).

In a third passage from the same chapter Locke believes himself to be elucidating the meaning of a "free agent" rather than of simply "an agent." In this he is, like many others both before and since, mistaken. For, as we have just seen, both those who act of their own free will and those who act under compulsion are equally agents, choosing to act as they actually do act rather than to act in any of the alternative ways that were in fact open to them at the time in question:

> We have instances enough, and often more than enough in our own bodies. A Man's Heart beats, and the Blood circulates, which 'tis not in his Power...to stop, and therefore in respect of these Motions, where rest depends not on his choice...he is not a *free agent*. Convulsive motions agitate his legs, so that though he will it never so much, he cannot...stop their motion (as in that odd disease called *Chorea Sancti Viti*[5] but he is moving as a Stone that falls or a Tennis-ball struck with a Racket (Locke [1690] 1975, II [xxi], p. 239).

With reminders of these three passages before us we are in a position to develop ostensive definitions of two contrasting kinds of bodily movements. Going deliberately with rather than against the grain of modern English usage, let those which can be either initiated or quashed at will be labelled "movings," and those which cannot "motions." Those active exercises of a "*Power* to begin or forbear" that in the first two of these three passages Locke called motions become movings, whereas the passive and uncontrollable motions described in the third passage, such as those occurring when "A Man's Heart beats and the Blood circulates" and "which 'tis not in his Power...to stop" all continue to be described as motions. Anyone exercising his or her "*Power* to begin or forbear" is thereby making a choice, and thus showing himself or herself to be an agent.

It is, therefore, in terms of the fundamental distinction between movings and motions that we become able to explicate the equally fundamental concept of action. An agent is a creature who, precisely and only in so far as he or she is an agent, can and cannot but make choices: choices between the alternative courses of action or inaction that are from time to time open to him or her as an individual; real choices between genuine alternative possibilities notwithstanding that sometimes by opting for even any one of these open alternatives the agents concerned would incur formidable costs. Agents, too, *qua* agents—it is the price of privilege—inescapably must choose, and can in no way avoid choosing, one of the two or usually many more options which on particular occasions are open and available to them. This is a point upon which Locke too had insisted in the same chapter as that from which the three previous quotations were taken:

> For it is unavoidably necessary to prefer the doing, or forbearance, of an Action in a Man's power, which is once so proposed to his thoughts; a Man must necessarily *will* the one, or the other of them, upon which preference, or volition, the action, or its forbearance, certainly follows, and is truly voluntary: But the act of volition, or preferring one of the two, being that which he cannot avoid, a Man in respect of that act of *willing*, is under a necessity (Locke [1690] 1975, II [xxi] 23, pp. 245-6).[6]

The next step, having elucidated the notions of being an agent, of having a choice, and of being able to do otherwise than in the event one actually does do, is first to distinguish two fundamentally different senses of the word "power" and then to show the sorts of universally available experience from which the ideas of physical (as opposed to logical) necessity and physical (as opposed to logical) impossibility can be derived.

In the first two passages quoted from Locke he was concerned exclusively with the sort of power that can be predicated only of people—or of such other putative, quasipersonal beings as the theist God, the Olypmian gods, archangels, angels, devils, and other assorted disembodied or ever-bodiless spirits. Let us, therefore, attach to this first sort of power the label "power (personal)." A power (personal) is an ability either to do or to abstain from doing whatever it may be.

In another sense, which is the only sense in which the word can be applied to inanimate objects and to most of animate nature, a power simply is a disposition to behave in such and such a way, given that such and such preconditions are satisfied. Thus we might say that the "nuclear device" dropped at Nagasaki possessed an explosive power equivalent to that of so many tons of TNT, or that full-weight nylon climbing rope has a breaking strain of (a power to hold up to) 4,500 pounds. Let us label this second sort of power "power (physical)."

It is in this third passage quoted from Locke that we find him indicating the kind of confrontations with physical necessities and physical impossibilities with which all human beings are inescapably familiar and from our experience of which our ideas of physical (as opposed to logical) necessities and physical (as opposed to logical) impossibilities could have and surely must have been derived.[7] These are the "instances enough, and often more than enough in our own bodies" in which "A Man's Heart beats, and the Blood circulates, which 'tis not in his Power...to stop" and the "Convulsive motions" of "that odd disease called *Chorea Sancti Viti*" in all of which cases their subject is "under as much Necessity of moving, as a Stone that falls or a Tennis-ball struck with a Rackett."

The importance of the complementary ideas thus derived lies in the fact that they are essential to the scientifically fundamental conception of a law of nature. That conception itself can perhaps best be illuminated by introducing the intellectually indispensable concept, not so far explicitly mentioned, of the contrary-to-fact conditional proposition.

A contrary-to-fact conditional is a proposition of the form: "If this were to have happened (which perhaps, as a matter of fact, it did not), then that would have occurred (which perhaps, as a matter of fact, it did not)." Such propositions are relevant and of great importance because nomologicals[8] (propositions stating what are thought to constitute laws of nature) can be distinguished from merely material implications (propositions stating—without any implications about what might have been but in fact was not—only not-as-a-matter-of-fact-this-and-not-that) by the logical fact that they entail contrary-to-fact conditionals. Also implicit in the notion of nomological is the idea of physical necessity. It is precisely and only because to assert that certain relationships between sorts of logically possible events hold with physical necessity that we become licensed to infer contrary-to-fact conditionals from nomologicals.

The whole preceding logical analysis of agency and of the several notions closely related to it shows very clearly that agents, *qua* agents—it is the price of privilege—inescapably must choose—can in no way avoid choosing—one of the two or usually many more options that on particular occasions are open and available to them. For the nerve of the distinction between the movings involved in an action and the motions that constitute no more than items or partial components of necessitated behavior is that such behavior is physically necessitated; whereas the sense, the direction, and the character of actions as such not merely is not as a matter of brute fact necessitated, but, as a matter of logic, necessarily cannot be.

It therefore becomes impossible to maintain the doctrine of universal physically necessitating determinism, the doctrine, that is to say, that every movement in the Universe—including every human bodily movement, the movings as well as the motions—is determined by physically necessitating physical causes. The most that can be allowed is that we are so determined to be people who will in fact choose to act in whatever senses we do in fact severally choose to act. Nevertheless, this said, we have at once to add that it is the previous choices of every individual that must play a large part in physically causing those individuals to be the people who will in fact make their several choices in whatever always physically unnecessitated particular senses they individually choose.

That should, surely, be sufficient to justify holding at least some individuals—why not *most*?—fully responsible for at least some of their actions—why not *most*? This is, of course, always providing that the buck really stops with them and that there is no other person, or quasi-personal Being, physically necessitating those individuals to be the people who do in fact choose in whatever senses they do choose.

But where does the Buck Actually Stop?[9]

That proviso "that the buck really stops with them" is of the last importance. For there is an enormous difference between, on the one hand, even an in principle predictable determination by entirely impersonal and unintending physical causes and, on the other hand, Divine predestination. But it would seem that, for the theist in the mainstream Judaeo-Christian and Islamic traditions,[10] that crucial proviso is not satisfied. Anyone not interested in either of those traditions should skip the present section.

Christians today typically think first of the relations between their God and His human creatures on the model of those between a human father and his children. No doubt it is true that it is only in certain scandalous and extremely exceptional cases that parents can properly be held responsible for the misdeeds of their grown-up children; and then, even in those rare cases, only partially and rather remotely. But in this aspect, which is here crucial, that preferred model is totally inapplicable. For if we were indeed creatures of a Creator in any traditional Judaeo-Christian or Islamic understanding, then, as the omnipotent and omniscient ultimate sustaining cause of everything that exists or happens within the supposedly created Universe, God must necessarily make us the various individual people who, confronted inescapably with choices to be made, do in fact choose as we do choose. Such a God must therefore, *ex hypothesi*, be the ultimately responsible necessitating cause of everything; and everything means everything, including all those sins for which unforgiven sinners are to be punished so unjustly and so inordinately by their Creator with extremes of unending torture.

To this the usual indignant response today is to protest that it is only hard, unfashionable Calvinists who believe in the predestination that carries such appalling implications. The rest instead insist that the Creator endowed human beings—"made in His own image"—with freewill; thus, they believe, ensuring that God is not responsible for our making the sinful choices we so perversely and persistently do make.

This response is on two accounts mistaken. It is mistaken, in the first place, because predestinationism—the doctrine, that is to say, that God predetermines the senses of the choices for which He holds the creatures making those choices fully accountable—is not in fact peculiar to Calvin and Calvinists. On the contrary it is, for a start, certainly Biblical. St. Paul had a first class philosophical mind. So he saw at once and without hesitation the logically necessary implications of maintaining that the Universe and everything and everyone in it was created and is sustained by an omnipotent and omniscient personal Being who nevertheless punishes creatures inordinately for delinquencies of which He himself is necessarily the necessitating cause:[11]

> For the scripture saith unto Pharaoh, Even for this same purpose have I raised thee up, that I might show my power in thee, and that my name might be declared throughout all the earth. Therefore hath he mercy upon whom he will have mercy, and whom he will he hardeneth. Thou wilt say then unto me, Why doth he yet find fault? For who hath resisted his will? Nay but, O man who art thou that repliest against God? Shall the thing formed say to him that formed it, Why hast thou made me thus? Hath not the potter the power over the clay, of the same lump to make one vessel unto honour and another unto dishonour? What if God, willing to show his wrath, and to make his power known, endured with much long suffering the vessels of wrath fitted to destruction; and that he might make known the riches of his glory on the vessels of mercy, which he had afore prepared unto glory, even us, whom he hath called, not of the Jews only but also of the Gentiles? (*Romans*, IX, 17-24).

Luther, to his credit, made clear during his controversy with Erasmus that he was appalled by these predestinarian implications. He nevertheless realized that they are inescapable:

> Common sense and natural reason are highly offended that God by his mere will deserts, hardens, and damns, as if delighted in sins and such eternal torments, he who is said to be of such mercy and goodness. Such concept of God appears wicked, cruel, and intolerable, and by it many men have been revolted in all ages. I myself was once offended to the very depth of the abyss of desperation, so that I wished I had never been created. There is no use trying to get away from this by ingenious distinctions. Natural reason, however much it is offended, must admit the consequences of the omniscience and omnipotence of God (E. G. Rupp et al. [eds.], 1969, p. 130).

Later, Luther addresses himself to the question: "Why then does He not alter those evil wills which He moves?" Understandably, if unsatisfactorily, Erasmus receives no answer:

> It is not for us to inquire into the mysteries, but to adore them. If flesh and blood take offence here and grumble, well, let them grumble; they will achieve nothing; grumbling will not change God! And however many of the ungodly stumble and depart, the elect will remain (Ibid., p. 130).

The not very near nearest which Luther comes to any solution to what he sees as of these mysteries is to appeal to faith:

> The highest degree of faith is to believe He is just, though of His own will he makes us…proper subjects for damnation, and seems (in the words of Erasmus) "to delight in the torments of poor wretches and to be a fitter object for hate than for love." If I could by any means understand how this same God…can yet be merciful and just, there would be no need for faith. (Ibid., p. 139).

Today many thoroughly instructed Roman Catholics may be surprised to learn that the same appalling doctrine of Divine predestination has been, and presumably still is, an essential element in their faith. Thus the *Summa Theologica* contains a Question "Of Predestination" in which the Angelic Doctor lays it down that:

> As men are ordained to eternal life through the providence of God, it likewise is part of that providence to permit some to fall away from that end; this is called reprobation… Reprobation implies not only foreknowledge but also is something more… (I [xxiii] 3).

What and how much that something more is the *Summa contra Gentiles* makes clear:

> …just as God not only gave being to things when they first began, but is also—as the conserving cause of being—the cause of their being as long as they last…so He also not only gave things their operative powers when they were first created, but is also always the cause of these in things. Hence if this divine influence stopped every operation would stop. Every operation therefore, of anything is traced back to Him as its cause (Book III, Chapter 67).

This is spelt out more fully in two later chapters:

> God alone can move the will, as an agent, without doing violence to it... Some people...not understanding how God can cause a movement of our will, have tried to explain...authoritative texts wrongly; that is, they would say that God "works in us, to wish and to accomplish" means that He causes in us the power of willing, but not in such a way that He makes us will this or that...these people are, of course, opposed quite plainly by authoritative texts of Holy Writ. For it says in *Isaiah* (xxxvi, 2) "Lord, you have worked all our work in us."[12] Hence we receive from God not only the power of willing but its employment also (Book III, Chapters 88-9).

The Angelic Doctor, however, is always the devotedly complacent apparatchik. He sees no problem about the justice of either the inflicting of infinite and everlasting penalties for finite and temporal offences or their inflicting upon creatures for offences that their Creator makes them (choose to) commit. For:

> In order that the happiness of the saints may be more delightful to them and that they may render more copious thanks to God...they are allowed to see perfectly the sufferings of the damned...the Divine Justice and their own deliverance will be the direct cause of the joy of the blessed, while the pains of the damned will cause it indirectly...the blessed in glory will have no pity for the damned (*Summa Theologica* III, Supp. [xciv] 1-3).[13]

There is a second reason why it is mistaken to insist that the Creator endowed human beings—"'made in His own image"—with free will, thus ensuring that God is not responsible for our making the sinful choices we so perversely and persistently do make.

This reason is that predestinationists do not in fact deny that we are members of a kind of creatures who can and therefore cannot but make choices, choices some of which are made by the agents of their own free will and some of which are made under various forms and degrees of coercion and constraint. If and so in so far as any predestinationists do deny free will it is only in some factitious misunderstanding of the word "freewill," a misunderstanding introduced in a vain attempt to refute the charge that the God of Judaeo-Christian and Islamic theism must be recognized as necessarily being one causally necessitating His creatures to choose—though free of any this worldly coercion or constraint—to do deeds for which He proposes to punish them with an eternity of torture. Luther had his own characteristically vehement way of dismissing this "freewill defence"[14] of Divine Justice:

> Now, by "necessarily" I do not mean compulsorily but by the necessity of immutability (as they say) and not of compulsion. That is to say, when a man is without the Spirit of God he does not do evil against his will, as if he were taken by the scruff of his neck and

forced to do it, like a thief or a robber carried off against his will to punishment, but he does it of his own accord and with a ready will (E. G. Rupp et al. [eds.], 1969, p. 139).

This present excursion into philosophical theology can, therefore, appropriately be concluded with a fifth and final quotation from that same great chapter "Of Power" in Locke's *Essay Concerning Human Understanding*:

> I leave it to be considered, whether it may not help to put an end to that long agitated, and, I think, unreasonable, because unintelligible, Question, viz. *Whether Man's Will be free or no*. For if I mistake not, it follows from what I have said, that the Question itself is altogether improper, and it is as insignificant to ask, whether Man's Will be free, as to ask, whether his Sleep be Swift, or his Vertue square...and when anyone well considers it, I think he will as plainly perceive, that *Liberty* which is but a power, belongs only to Agents, and cannot be an attribute or modification of the Will, which is also but a *Power* (Locke [1690] 1975, II [xxi] 14, p. 240).

Notes

1. See for instance, for the UK, Dennis and Erdos 1992 plus Hitchens 1999, and for the USA, Bork 1996.
2. Compare "Thou Shalt Not Commit a Value Judgement," Chapter 1 of Dennis and Erdos 1992.
3. *Growth and Inflation* (London: Church Information office, 1975), pp. 1-2. For more and more recent evidence of the decline in that church both of commitment to essentials of the traditional Christian faith and of emphasis upon individual responsibility compare Chapter 4, below.
4. For a more exhaustive critique of this particular work see Flew 1978, chapter 7.
5. The Latin translates as "St. Vitus' dance."
6. As the existentialist Jean-Paul Sartre famously said: "Not to choose is, in effect, to choose not to choose" (Sartre, 1957, p. 481).
7. For attempts to show that these are the "impressions" from which Hume could and indeed should have derived the complementary "ideas" of physical necessity and physical impossibility see my "What Impressions of Necessity" in *Hume Studies*, Vol.XVIII, No. 2 (1992), or "The Legitimation of Factual Necessity" in Macintosh, J. J. and Meynell, H. A. (eds.), *Faith, Scepticism and Personal Identity* (Calgary: Calgary University Press, 1994), or "Second Thoughts about the *First Enquiry*" in *Philosophical Writings*, No. 10 (Spring 1999).
8. "Nomos" is the Greek word for law.
9. Some may like to be informed or reminded that President Truman had a notice on the desk of his office in the White House to remind him that "The buck stops here."
10. For the relevance here of that tradition see "The Terrors of Islam," chapter 20 in Kurtz, Paul (ed.), *Challenges to the Enlightenment* (Buffalo, NY: Prometheus, 1994).
11. Those who know of the Church of England only in its present (in more than one sense) secular decline will perhaps be surprised to learn that once upon a time its Commission on Doctrine unhesitatingly affirmed "that the whole course of events is under the control of God," and appreciated that "logically this involves the affirmation of that there is no event, and no aspect of any event, even those due to sin and

so contrary to the Divine will, which falls outside the scope of his purposive activity" (*Doctrine in the Church of England*, London, 1922, p. 47).

12. Aquinas chose an Old Testament rather than New Testament text because the *Summa contra Gentiles* was directed towards Muslims.
13. As used to be said in my day in the unhallowed ranks of the Royal Air Force, "F... you, Jack, I'm fireproof."
14. For a critique of this defense, as employed by C. S. Lewis, surely the most persuasive Christian apologist of the second half of the twentieth century, see Flew and MacIntyre (eds.), 1955, chapter VIII.

3

State Welfare and Individual Demoralization

I am deeply convinced that any permanent, regular, administrative system whose aim will be to provide for the needs of the poor, will breed more miseries than it can cure, will deprave the population that it wants to help and comfort...will dry up the source of savings, will stop the accumulation of capital, will retard the development of trade and will benumb human industry and activity.—Alexis de Tocqueville, Memoir on Pauperism *(1835)*

A welfare state, for present purposes, is one in which very extensive health and educational services are provided, in which there is also very extensive provision of financial and other forms of support for those deemed unable adequately to provide for themselves and their dependents, and in which by far the greater part of all this provision is financed out of taxation either immediate or, in the shape of government borrowing, deferred. In this understanding, all the member countries of the OECD (Organisation for Economic Cooperation and Development) must be accounted as being or having developed, if not overdeveloped, welfare states. But here we shall be considering only the United Kingdom, with occasional glances across the Atlantic to the United States.

Many, if not most or even all, of these first world countries have growing difficulties in meeting escalating financial demands from their welfare states—demands that tend to divert to present consumption resources that should in prudence be devoted to productive investment promising future returns. The two main causes of these increased financial demands are increases in the numbers and proportions of their total populations becoming and remaining entitled to support from what are apparently always unfunded state pension schemes, and increases in the numbers and proportions of the remainder of these total populations becoming and remaining entitled to various other state provided welfare benefits.

What the Welfare State Crowded Out

As in so many other cases, here too what Edmund Burke would have described as "very plausible" and "very pleasing commencements" have led on to "shameful and lamentable conclusions." However, before we consider conclusions consequent upon continuing to maintain a comprehensive welfare state, we need to notice some of the worthy and desirable practices and institutions which, through its establishment, were inevitably either diminished or destroyed.

For instance, before the passage of the 1870 Forster Education Act began the process eventually leading to today's monopolistic state-maintained school system, there was in the UK extraordinarily extensive private provision of primary education.[1] Here, however, we will be concerned primarily with the tax-financed provision of financial and other forms of support for those deemed unable adequately to provide for themselves and/or their dependents. We shall be concerned, that is to say, with what Americans would naturally describe as being itself, without qualification, the welfare state.

Before the passage of the 1911 National Insurance Act, which laid the first foundations for the construction in Britain after World War II of both the National Health Service and a comprehensive welfare system, there was in these areas also a vast and steadily increasing amount of voluntary effort. This was both voluntary charitable effort and voluntary effort to provide by mutual aid much of what was later to be provided entirely or almost entirely by the state. By the time that under that act the government had introduced compulsory social insurance for 12 million persons "at least 9 million were already covered by registered and unregistered voluntary insurance associations, chiefly the friendly societies,"[2] and "the rate of growth over the preceding thirty years had been accelerating."[3]

Before 1911, a variety of friendly society providers, often locally administered by their own volunteer members, competed to serve their members both better and more economically. Their achievement was accepted as a model by Lloyd George, who piloted the 1911 National Insurance Act through Parliament. Indeed, he originally saw the bill that eventually became this act as a means of extending the benefits of friendly society membership to the entire employed population.

However, the combined opposition both of the organized medical profession, which had always resented the dominance of the largely working class medical consumer, and of the trade association of the commercial insurance companies, which had suffered from the competition of the non-profit friendly societies, succeeded in introducing very substantial amendments. In sum, these both crowded out the friendly societies and ensured that, through its implementation of the resulting act, "the Government nearly doubled doctors' incomes," whereas previously "doctors' pay had been kept within limits that ordinary manual workers could afford."[4]

Locally administered and voluntary friendly societies were also better able than centralized bureaucracies to diminish "moral hazard" in the form of fraudulent or otherwise improper acquisitions of benefits. Whereas the Prudential Assurance Company had had to abandon the provision of sick pay because, as its Secretary told the Royal Commission on Friendly Societies in 1873, "after five years' experience we found that we were unable to cope with the fraud that was practised," the friendly societies found that not only was effective supervision more feasible, but it was also possible to create a real sense of moral responsibility among members. Those who chose to cheat were defrauding not some huge and remote collective but their own immediate associates. For the funds of each branch were all and only the contributions of each member. To apply for sick pay members had to obtain a certificate of disability from the lodge doctor, and these claims were considered at the monthly branch meetings. Nor was sick pay paid automatically for every sort of sickness regardless of the individual's responsibility for suffering that affliction: "Most societies, for instance, had rules which excluded indisposition due to venereal disease or drunkenness."[5]

Social Laws and "Social" Justice

All inquiry into the "shameful and lamentable conclusions" that may follow from the development of a state welfare system has to start from a recognition of the logically necessary truth of the Law of Unintended Rewards. This, as originally formulated in 1980 by Charles Murray, states that "Any social transfer increases the net value of being in the condition that prompted the transfer." Many, if not all, of those involved in the establishment and maintenance of state welfare systems have been well aware that numerous conditions unintentionally "rewarded" by such systems are conditions into which at least some of their victims could and surely ought to have avoided falling and/or which they could and surely ought to escape partly or wholly by their own efforts. In the UK, however, the "moral neutrality" that was later to be justified by reference to the doctrine of anti-social determinism was actually required by the 1911 National Insurance Act. It was that Act of Parliament that originally established that which was subsequently to grow into the enormous, not to say monstrous,[6] British welfare state. In that very different earlier period the deserving poor and the deserving no-so-poor were generally characterized by a self-reliant resolve never to accept charity. It was therefore necessary to show that benefits under the 1911 National Insurance Act would be financed at least in large part from premia paid by the beneficiaries, since these benefits were intended to be seen by their beneficiaries not as charity but as property which was already justly and of right theirs.[7]

In the years since there have been two relevant developments. There have, first, been universal, European, and other declarations of human rights that have included welfare as well as option rights. Option rights, like those proclaimed in the American Declaration of Independence, are the rights of individuals to be left to their own devices, provided only that they respect the equal rights of others. Welfare rights are rights to be provided with some sort of good, necessarily at the expense of others and presumably by the appropriate organ of the local welfare state.

There has, second, been an enormous increase in the prevalence of talk about social justice, or—taking these two ideals to be necessarily connected if not actually equivalent—about equality and social justice. It is perhaps well to remind ourselves of how comparatively recent this increase has been. For in the English language the earliest employment of the expression "social justice" recorded by the revisers of the *Oxford English Dictionary* occurs in 1861, in chapter V of J. S. Mill's *Utilitarianism*. In Italian it has been found considerably earlier. Very reasonably the finder remarked: "We should all have been spared a good deal of muddleheadedness if Taparelli, who coined the expression in the 1840s, had bothered to tell us what he meant by it."

For many years thereafter almost everyone employing the expression "social justice" followed Taparelli in not bothering to tell us what they meant by it. This was, for instance, conspicuously true of the author of a work called *Elements of Social Justice* widely recommended to students for twenty-five or more years after its first publication in 1922.[8] In that book the expression "social justice" is actually employed only once, and without explanation, on the very first page of the text. At this stage—before we proceed, in chapter five below, to provide a more radical critique—the expression "social justice" can perhaps be defined most illuminatingly as referring to what is or would be produced by the operations of an ideal welfare system and the massive and steeply progressive taxation required for its support. Certainly that is how the British Labour party's "independent" Commission on Social Justice, which reported towards the end of 1994, construed its terms of reference.

Indeed, this ideal of equality and social justice is perhaps best conceived as the justifying ideology of the welfare state and of all those who today claim the social democratic name (or in the USA that of liberal or left-liberal Democrat). For it provides the rationale not only for the state monopoly provision of health, education, and welfare services but also for the maximum possible transfers through the tax and welfare systems from the better-off to the worse-off. The consequent relativistic definitions of poverty as a substantial falling below the average income, however high that average income may become, guarantee the permanent continuation of perceived needs for ever more purportedly poverty-relieving state handouts.[9]

The operation of the Law of Unintended Rewards is one main cause of the expansion in the numbers of those becoming and remaining entitled to various welfare state benefits. It is remarkable that Milton Friedman—of all people—in presenting his proposals for a negative income tax (NIT), seems never to have considered the relevance to its introduction of the economists' general Law of Supply and Demand, from which Murray was later to formulate his Law of Unintended Rewards. For, as we may learn from Murray 1984, pp. 148-53, it was in an attempt to meet the objection that the introduction of such a guaranteed income would cause people to reduce their work effort or to drop out of the labor force altogether that the Office of Economic Opportunity set up "the most ambitious social-science experiment in history." The result was totally decisive, demonstrating unequivocally that the objectors had been right.

Another main cause of the expansion in the numbers of those becoming and remaining entitled to various welfare benefits is the admission of fundamental human rights to welfare. Once one or two moral rights of this kind have been admitted there seems to be no rational stopping point. Such an admission opens the way to an indefinite extension of the diversity of the benefits that allegedly ought to be made available. Making such supposedly moral rights also legal entitlements is then seen as the imperative demand of "social" justice.

It may perhaps be allowed, as Hayek himself conceded in *The Mirage of Social Justice*, that "There is no reason why in a free society government should not assure to all protection against severe deprivation in the form of an assured minimum income, a floor below which nobody needs to descend."[10] A prudent and restrained government would, however, even when that assured minimum income was to be absolutely low, still—at least in the case of conditions that could have been or could now be avoided—try to find ways of channelling any necessary tax-financed assistance through private organizations better able and more inclined than any centralized state bureaucracy effectively to distinguish deserving from undeserving recipients.

As Hayek always insisted, the mischievous idea that all public needs should be satisfied by compulsory organization "is wholly alien to the basic principles of a free society. The true liberal must on the contrary desire as many as possible of those particular societies within the state, voluntary organizations between the individual and government, which...Rousseau and the French Revolution wanted to suppress."[11]

The effects of the operation of the Law of Unintended Rewards are bound to be stronger and more widespread to the extent that poverty is relatively defined. To some extent it no doubt always has been and has to be, but the recent dissociation of the idea of poverty from traditional conceptions involving "severe deprivation" and actual hardship generates wildly paradoxical implications once we begin to make comparisons between the actual material conditions of those rated as poor at different times, in different places, and by different standards.[12]

Those who have memories of the actual material conditions of those in the United Kingdom who were unemployed and dependent upon the available state-provided benefits during the 1930s find it hard to believe that the operation of the Law of Unintended Rewards produced substantial effects during that period. Yet a 1992 study unambiguously revealed the extent of the effects of what to us today must seem the extremely modest increases which were made in 1920 in the amounts and the availability of unemployment benefits:

> In summary, the cross-sectional evidence...reveals a pattern that is inescapable; the inter-war unemployment system importantly shaped the unemployment histories of every nook and cranny of Britain. Whether one examines the pattern of age, sex, industry, duration, location, or skill, one simple fact emerges: lowering the cost of an activity (or inactivity) induces more of that activity (or inactivity). In the present instance, lowering the cost of unemployment induced more unemployment in inter-war Britain.[13]

The effects of the unintended rewards for unemployment provided by social transfer programs may be and in fact are increased by any reductions in the rewards actually provided by any available forms of employment. In large part because of the increasing percentages of GDP required to meet the ever rising costs of the welfare state, the proportions of below average incomes taken by taxation have vastly increased in recent decades, certainly in the United Kingdom but perhaps not in the United States.

Thus, for example, an earlier study (Hermione Parker 1982) had found that in the United Kingdom persons earning half the national average income paid 25 percent of their earnings in tax and national insurance contributions, which was more than single people earning *twice* the national average income had been paying in 1950 (p. 73). Again, in 1950, at national average earnings, a two-child family paid just under 4 percent of their total income (earnings plus family allowances) in national insurance contributions and income tax, whereas a four-child family paid 3 percent of its income in national insurance contributions *and no income tax at all*. Between 1950 and 1981, the tax burden for the two-child family increased to 26 percent of total income, but during the same thirty-one-year period the four-child family was drawn into the income tax net, and their tax burden increased *eightfold* to 24 percent (Ibid., p. 73).

During the same period, inevitably, the *net* reward for lower-paid forms of work began to compare unfavorably with the total package of benefits during unemployment, with a consequent tendency for the total of those officially unemployed to increase. All this was bound to have various general effects on the economy. When, for instance, "as in Britain, the net rewards for skilled and semi-skilled work are only marginally higher than the net rewards for unskilled work, then vacancies for skilled labour (become) difficult to fill. Labour shortages...then co-exist alongside apparently high unemployment" (Ibid., p. 25).

The extent of consequent demoralization in the labor force is not of course revealed by any official statistics. We can do no more than guesstimate how many of those registered and continuing to draw benefits as unemployed are either regularly supplementing these benefits with earnings in the black economy or have effectively lost any desire to support themselves and any dependents from their own earnings, whether legitimate or illegitimate.

An important special case of unintended rewards for what is perhaps not, strictly speaking, registered unemployment is the abuse of the incapacity benefit system. As with all questions related to the black economy it is impossible to produce accurate statistics. But there can be no doubt but that a very large number of those drawing incapacity benefit are no longer truly entitled to do so. For shortly after Prime Minister Blair announced that new legislation would require the cases of all persons drawing this kind of benefit to be medically reviewed every three years a pseudonymous but in fact well known medical doctor asserted in a serious London weekly that "The number of people claiming incapacity benefit has tripled since 1980, to 2.3 million."[14]

He went on to ask "Are there really 2.3 million people of working age in this country who are too ill to work? Is it that we were hard-hearted in 1980 and forced people to work who were, strictly speaking, unable to do so?" Having asked the question he gave his own confident answer:

> Every doctor in the country knows that a very high percentage of the people on incapacity benefit either have no real illness at all, or an illness that is certainly not incapacitating except to those who do not wish to work. Sickness notes are signed by doctors because of threats of unpleasant scenes in their surgeries, or even in violence towards them, not because of ascertainable illness. What is more, the whole fraudulent process is encouraged by the gradual redefinition of patterns of bad behaviour as bona fide illnesses. Even persistent lying about being ill has now been defined as an illness. In other words, you are sick if you think—or claim—that you are.

Dr. Dalrymple's first comment is that "This is all a manifestation of the great cultural movement away from making a judgement about personal desert and its opposite," something we are bound to see as, at least in part, consequent upon the spread of the doctrine of anti-social determinism.

In the following sections we move into that area of the welfare system in which the operation of the Law of Unintended Rewards, powerfully reinforced both by general contemporary social tendencies and by particularly short-sighted changes in the taxation and legal systems, is in the UK having the most dramatic and irreparably damaging effects.

The Rise of Single Motherhood and the Decline of the Family

Any increase in unemployment matters, and anything that induces anyone to prefer dependent idleness to working for a living constitutes an affront to the ideals of a classically liberal Great Society.[15] By far and away the most devastating of all the demoralizing unintended rewards offered by welfare payments are those that encourage never-married single motherhood and the consequent growth of an underclass of what our Victorian forebears would not have hesitated to rate as the undeserving poor. The members of such a class, which has a strong tendency to reproduce itself, are characterized by the rejection of all the traditional norms governing the behavior of the deserving poor. The most comprehensive and well-evidenced account of the development of such an underclass, and of the part played in this development by the unintended rewards offered in welfare payments, comes from the United States and was provided by Charles Murray.[16]

It is important to insist that the part played in such developments by the unintended rewards presented by the welfare system is by no means the only part. Indeed, it should be altogether obvious that the explosive growth of never-married single motherhood cannot be understood except in the context of vast increases in premarital and extramarital sexual activity, of divorce, of the consequent father-absent upbringing of the children of those broken marriages, and of several other negative social phenomena as well. Nor would it be sensible to attempt to produce a policy for dealing with the problem of never-married motherhood by attending only to the perverse incentives provided by the welfare system, and without taking account of all those other contextual factors.

It was apparently attention to all the relevant factors in United States society as a whole which, in that country, eventually persuaded "politicians of all ideological persuasions...that *only* family reconstruction can save the nation from social disaster."[17] Unfortunately, that is most certainly not the case in the United Kingdom. For here many professing social scientists and social policy pundits bigotedly persist in ignoring

> the findings of research on the life chances of the child from the family where both parents were married when the child was born, and where both parents successfully struggled to stay together to look after it. The life chances of such a child are on the average better than those of the child from any other situation of conception and child-rearing that is at all possible on a large scale, and much better than the child from the father-absent situation.[18]

Life chances here embrace the likelihoods of dying in infancy, of becoming criminally delinquent, of underachieving in education, and of just about every other negative outcome a social scientist could think of measuring. Of course, like almost all the findings of the social sciences, these refer to likelihoods and averages. It is, therefore, both possible and common to hear people claiming to have rubbished them by citing—as we all can—individual instances of unsuccessful parenting by some devoted married couples and/or of successful parenting by some never-married mother. But when such pseudo-refutations are offered—as I myself have certainly heard them offered—by persons with social scientific pretensions, then they ought to be construed as tacit and unwilling admissions of an inability to point to even one piece of quantitative research contradicting the consensus "of every empirical study that has ever been published on the subject that has yielded definite results on the benefits and drawbacks of families with fathers as compared to those households without them."[19]

In the United Kingdom as in the United States growing numbers of marital separations and divorces were at one time almost the sole cause of increases in the numbers of lone-parent households and in the numbers of dependent children living in such households. The increases in all these numbers during the last quarter-century have been formidable. During that period there has in addition been not only a huge and altogether unprecedented increase in the number of never-married mothers but also, in consequence, an increase in their proportion in the totals of lone-parent households.

Thus, the number of lone-parent households in the United Kingdom more than doubled between 1971 and 1991, as did the number of children living in such households, while between 1961 and 1991 the percentage of all those living in such households, multiplied four-fold (from 2.5 percent to 10 percent). Until 1984, nearly three-quarters of these increases was due to the growth in the numbers of divorced and separated mothers, and, as rates of remarriage have fallen during the seventies and the eighties, this has increased the contribution of rising divorce rates to the growth in the numbers of lone-parent households and of the dependent children contained therein.[20]

However, whereas in 1971 never-married mothers formed the smallest of all categories of lone parents with dependent children, by 1991 they formed the largest.[21] For, since the late seventies the number of births occurring outside marriage has been growing with unprecedented speed. In little over a decade, the rate rose from roughly one in ten to 31 percent in 1992, and it is continuing to rise at about 2 percent a year. For births to women under twenty years old, it has reached 84 percent. But even for births to women over thirty-five it was in 1991 a fifth, compared with a tenth in 1982.[22] A recent historical study makes clear just how unprecedented this situation is:

> The present illegitimacy ratio is not only unprecedented in the past two centuries; it is unprecedented, so far as we know, in American history going back to colonial times, and in English history from Tudor times. The American evidence is scanty, but the English is more conclusive. The English parish records in the mid-sixteenth century give an illegitimacy ratio of 2.4 per cent; by the early seventeenth century it reached 3.4 per cent; in the Cromwellian period it fell to one per cent; during the eighteenth century it rose from 3.1 per cent to 5.3 per cent; it reached its peak at 7 per cent in 1845, and then declined to under 4 per cent by the end of the nineteenth century. It is against this background that the present rate of over 30 percent must be viewed.[23]

The increasing *absolute numbers* of births outside marriage have to be explained exclusively by reference to changes in the relations between the various incentives to unmarried motherhood and the various disincentives against it. But a considerable part of the explanation of the increases in the *proportions* of all births which are births outside marriage is to be found in the combination of falling marriage rates and of falling birth rates within marriages. It is clear that these falling rates of intramarital birth and even of marriage are themselves in part a generally unintended consequence of something already mentioned above; namely, an enormous relative increase in the burden of taxation imposed upon married couples, especially married couples with dependent children, as opposed to the burden imposed upon couples of single people without parental responsibilities.

Charity compels us to concede that these predictable consequences were generally unintended. Yet realism requires the recognition that they were and remain among the policy objectives of various officially sponsored and publicly financed lobbying organizations.[24] For instance, the National Council for One Parent Families, one of the most effective of such organizations in Britain, supports the moves to abolish the tax allowance for the married, sees "no justification" for removing it from lone parents, and wants them to receive a lone-parent tax allowance in addition to ordinary child benefits, while a two-parent family enjoys only the ordinary child benefit.

What is to be Done?

In face of the overwhelming evidence of the far inferior parenting performance of lone-parent as opposed to two-parent families—evidence that certainly cannot be entirely or even mainly explained away by referring to the comparative poverty of lone-parent families[25]—it might seem obvious that it ought to be a prime objective of social policy to reduce both the numbers of such families and the proportion that they represent in the total of all families. Against this it is often objected that to formulate such a policy is to refuse to accept ineluctable realities: "It is like having a weather policy which instead of providing umbrellas tries to stop the rain from falling."[26] The fundamental reality that distinguishes the subject matter of the human from that of the physical sciences is, as we have been insisting from the beginning, that we are all examples of a kind of creature that can and cannot but make choices. Both lone-parent and two-parent families result from choices made by the two biological parents. These choices can be and in fact ultimately always are socially influenced—are influenced, that is to say, by what ultimately is itself always and only the verbal and non-verbal behavior of other individuals. So there is, in principle, nothing more unrealistic about policies to discourage the formation of one-parent families or to encourage the formation of two-parent families than there is in policies to induce people to change their diet, to stop smoking, or to eschew alcoholic drinks before driving motor vehicles.

In view of all this it should be astonishing and even scandalizing to find that the director of that leading British social science institution, the London School of Economics, a man whom Prime Minister Blair, while he himself was still only Leader of the Opposition, acknowledged as his guru, responded, when confronted with divorce rates of 40 percent or more, the explosive growth of single motherhood, and so on, by telling us that here "We are dealing with profound processes of change in everyday life, which it is well beyond the capacity of any political agency to reverse."[27]

Giddens was, in his book *The Third Way: The Renewal of Social Democracy* (Giddens 1998), attempting to develop policies suitable for a Labour Party which—otherwise despairing of ever again winning a Parliamentary majority in a General Election—had at very long last abandoned the socialist Clause IV of its original Constitution. This clause, which had for decades been printed on every Membership Card, stated simply that the ultimate objective of the Party was to achieve "the public ownership of all the means of production, distribution and exchange."

In discussing policy for the family Giddens starts encouragingly, asserting that "the family is a basic institution of civil society."[28] One might, however, have wished that he could have brought himself to recognize that the family is not "a" but *the* basic institution of civil society. Supposedly seeing "family policy" as "a key test for the new politics," Giddens proceeds to provide a potpourri of statistics from various member countries of the European Union, concluding from this that "In many countries only a minority of children are now brought up in a 'traditional' context where father and mother are married and living in the same household as their biological children, where the father is the economic breadwinner and the mother a housewife."[29]

We need to note the significant fact that for Giddens, the adjective "traditional" has here to be encased in what philosophers of my generation used to characterise as sneer quotes. Referring to the explosions of divorce, single motherhood, unmarried partnerships, and so on—which have "in many countries" produced a situation in which "only a minority of children are now brought up in a 'traditional' context"—Giddens proceeds to tell us that:

> The Right has a particular story to tell about the consequences of these changes: the family is in crisis because the traditional family is disintegrating. The remedies proposed flow from this analysis. The sanctity of marriage should be reaffirmed. Marriage is the main emotional training ground for errant males, binding them into duties and

> responsibilities they would otherwise abandon. Fatherlessness, according to such a view, "is the most harmful demographic trend of this generation... It is also the engine driving our most urgent social problems from crime to adolescent pregnancy to child sexual abuse to domestic violence against women..." Welfare measures that encourage single-parent households should be reformed to remove this effect.[30]

In quoting the above paragraph, three of the final four sentences have been omitted because they would appear to have been included in the original simply in order to distract attention from the subsequent demand for the reform of "Welfare measures that encourage single-parent households." For Giddens, the first step in opposing any such proposals is to present his readers with an extremely unattractive picture of what it is he wants to describe as the traditional family. The question of the faithfulness or otherwise of this picture of the English family up to the nineteenth and on into the first half of the twentieth century is, however, here irrelevant. For Giddens only introduces it in order unfairly to discredit what he dismisses as Rightist opposition before proceeding ungraciously to admit "that when today Rightist critics speak of the traditional family, they don't in fact mean" what Giddens here wants to describe as "the traditional family."[31]

His next step is not so much as even to mention, much less actually to examine, any of the published evidence and argument offered in support of proposals for the reform of "Welfare measures that encourage the growth of single-parent households" and the growth of various consequential phenomena. Instead it is, for Giddens and his intended readers, apparently sufficient simply to assert that these proposals came from "The Right" and, for that reason alone, to dismiss all the evidence and argument presented in support of those proposals. In thus refusing to examine evidence relevant to "our most urgent social problems" for no other or better reason than that that evidence is presented by chosen political opponents, *The Third Way* reveals itself as not only bigoted and obscurantist but also as frivolous.

But are these chosen opponents correctly described as coming exclusively from "The Right?" Certainly most of the relevant social scientific material has been published by the Health and Welfare Unit of the Institute of Economic Affairs, and certainly too *The Guardian* and *The Independent* insist on describing that Institute as a "rightwing think-tank." But it is not mere verbal trifling to point out that when in 1993 Norman Dennis and George Erdos' *Families without Fatherhood* was first published it contained a strongly endorsing Foreword by the lifelong socialist Professor A. H. Halsey. In that Foreword Halsey wrote:

> I share with my colleague Norman Dennis the value position of the ethical socialist as set out in our *English Ethical Socialism* (Oxford University Press, 1988). Central to that position is the doctrine of personal responsibility under virtually all social circumstances. People act under favourable and unfavourable conditions but remain responsible moral agents (p. xi).

Halsey then went on to insist that:

> What should be universally acknowledged is that the children of parents who do not follow the traditional norm (i.e. taking on personal, active and long-term responsibility for the social upbringing of the children they generate) are thereby disadvantaged in many major aspects of their chances of living a successful life. On the evidence available such children tend to die earlier, to have more illness, to do less well at school, to exist at a lower level of nutrition, comfort and conviviality, to suffer more unemployment, to be more prone to deviance and crime, and finally to repeat the cycle of unstable parenting from which they themselves have suffered (p. xiii).

The reasons why this should be universally acknowledged are, first, that it is of enormous social importance and, second, that the evidence that it is true is altogether decisive. The main reason why it is not universally acknowledged is that there appears to be among most of our professional social scientists and of our social affairs intellectuals what Dennis and Erdos have described as a *trahision des clercs*, a gritty determination to defend their own lifestyles by ignoring or ridiculing evidence pointing to the superiority of the traditional family.

As Dennis and Erdos themselves say, that determination "flies in the face of every empirical study that has ever been published on the subject which has yielded definite results on the benefits and drawbacks of families with fathers as opposed to those households without them."[32] Dennis went on in the following year to produce *Rising Crime and the Dismembered Family*, a work significantly subtitled *How Conformist Intellectuals Have Campaigned Against Common Sense*. He was remarkably well qualified to insist that there has indeed been a vast, not to say catastrophic, decline in the civility of the English people, from what we were before World War II and up until the nineteen fifties, to what we have since become. For he had been born in Sunderland before that war and when he later returned to research there he knew what the explosion in the criminal statistics meant. He knew better than to dismiss them—as many professing sociologists used to do in the columns of *New Society*—as if they were somehow mere expressions of a "moral panic."[33]

So let us now, after that digression along The Third Way, return to the contention that measures that promote never-married motherhood ought to be reformed. The fundamental objection to never-married motherhood is that never-married mothers produce children possessed of life chances substantially inferior to those that would have been enjoyed by their children had they given birth within the bonds of a stable marriage. What is meant here by inferior life chances is that the children of never-married mothers are more likely than the children of a stable marriage to become delinquent, more likely to underachieve educationally, and so on. But the children whom never-married mothers have actually produced serve them as hostages—their security against penalization.[34] Never-married motherhood is for this and many other reasons an extraordinarily difficult problem.

Yet it is, surely, beyond dispute that there can be little hope of halting the increase in never-married motherhood, much less of reversing the trend, until and unless the welfare state stops offering incentives and removing disincentives. For this is what it is now doing by providing various benefits both in cash and in kind, and by providing these as a matter of "social" justice and hence of both legal and moral right. If and in so far as, in the interests of the paradigmatically innocent children, state aid is necessary, then this should be routed via private charities, uninhibited by any calls to be "non-judgemental" and hence in effect tacitly approving of the mothers.

There is also a great deal that could be done to strengthen the institution of the two-parent two-sex family. In the first place, it is essential to reverse all those developments in the tax system and in the complementary welfare system which have had in combination the effect of making it much harder for married couples with low total family incomes to support children while making it much easier for single mothers to do so. The crux, as *The Times* (London) editorialized on November 10, 1993, is a very simple and straightforward "statistical fact: the sudden enormous increase in never-married mothers coincided with changes in the social welfare structure which rewarded that group preferentially over married couples."

The second major policy shift now needed to strengthen the institution of the family is to restore the support traditionally given to that most fundamental and important of social institutions.[35] In recent decades so many changes had been made in the laws of marriage and divorce having the effect of reducing that support, that by 1980 it was possible for one of the UK Law Commissioners to say that "logically we have already reached a point at which...we should be considering whether the legal institution of marriage continues to serve any useful purpose."[36] Whatever consideration followed within the Law Commission itself cannot have been either extensive or exhaustive, for in its 1988 report the Commission concluded that there was no reason why the legal system should support marriage in preference to "any other living arrangements."

It would surely be hard to find any precedents for such a conclusion in earlier legal literature. Consider, for instance, how in 1888, in its judgement in *Maynard v. Hill* (125 U.S. 190, 1888), the Supreme Court of the United States ruled that "other contracts may be modified, restricted or enlarged, or entirely released upon the consent of the parties. Not so with marriage... It is an institution, the purity of which the public is deeply interested in, for it is the foundation of the family and society without which there would be neither civilization nor any progress." That court went on to add that the obligations of marriage "arise not from the consent of concurring minds, but are the creation of the law itself: a relation the most important, as affecting the happiness of individuals, the first step from barbarism to incipient civilization, the purest tie of social life and the basis of human progress."

Contrast with the words of the British Law Commission the emphatic testimony of the anthropologist Bronislaw Malinowski. He more than once asserted that he could find no instance in the anthropological literature falsifying "the generalization: that in all human societies moral tradition and the law decree that the group consisting of a woman and her offspring is not a socially complete unit. The ruling of culture runs here. ...*[It] declares that the human family must consist of a male as well as a female*."[37] Of course, this generalization embraces the brief and recent period covered by historical and anthropological investigations; all but only the actual survivors, that is to say. But presumably they were, at least in an evolutionary biological sense, the fittest to survive.

Notes

1. Just how extensive this voluntary provision was can be learnt from Edwin G. West's *Education and the State: A Study in Political Economy* and from the same author's *Education and the Industrial Revolution*. Anyone challenging the characterization of the UK's state-maintained school system as monopolistic should be asked whether they can mention any anti-monopoly legislation anywhere in the world which would not be activated well before a single supplier controlled over 92 percent of the market; and even that is to take no account of the fact that that particular monopoly supplier has from the beginning operated a consistent policy of predatory not-pricing!
2. Green, David G., 1993, pp. 31-2.
3. Ibid., p .31.
4. Ibid., p. 98. We have here a remarkable confirming instance for Friedman's Law: "Everything government does costs twice as much."
5. Green 1993, p. 57.
6. The British National Health Service alone now, since the dissolution of the Red Army as such, vies with the Indian National Railways for the unenviable title of Worlds' Largest Employer.
7. For supposed Scriptural warrant for this doctrine see chapter 4, below.
8. This book by L. T. Hobhouse was indeed so recommended to me as an undergraduate at Oxford in the later 1940s.
9. See here Dennis, Norman, *The Invention of Permanent Poverty* (London: IEA Health and Welfare Unit, 1997). In this work Dennis, an ethical socialist and long time member of the Labour Party, takes as his target the almost universally acclaimed 1995 *Joseph Rowntree Foundation Inquiry into Income and Wealth* and, using the very same official statistical sources as are used by the poverty lobbies, reveals the manoeuvres that their members employ to substantiate their false claims.
10. Hayek 1976, p. 87.
11. Ibid., pp. 150-1. For a critical development of these Hayekian ideas, see Flew, Antony, "Social Justice Promotes Individual Dependency," in the *Journal of Libertarian Studies*, Vol. 11, No. 2, pp. 76-93.
12. For a challenging consideration of the way in which "equality and social justice" seems always to be an ideal (not of socialism but) of "equality and social justice" in one country, see Tullock, Gordon, "Patriotic Egalitarianism" in G. Radnitsky and H. Bouillon (eds.), *Values and the Social Order*, Vol. 2 (Aldershot: Avebury, 1995).
13. Matthews, Kent and Benjamin, Dan, 1994, *US and UK Unemployment between the Wars: A Doleful Story,* p. 110.
14. This and the subsequent quotations are from Dr. Theodore Dalrymple in *The Spectator* (London) for July 29, 2001.
15. For the greatest restatement of these ideals in a period of their decline, see Hayek, F.A., 1960, *The Constitution of Liberty*. For a more recent restatement compare Conway, David, 1995, *Classical Liberalism: The Unvanquished Ideal.*
16. Murray 1984. The same author has since deployed radical proposals for dealing with the problem in Murray 1998. He has also extended his inquiries to the United Kingdom, publishing his appropriately tentative findings along with much more categorical and often hostile British commentaries in Murray 1990 and Murray 1994.
17. Davies, Jon (ed.), 1993, p. 45 (emphasis original). This conclusion is supported by referring to the Final Report of the US National Commission on Children (Washington DC: US Government Printing Office, 1991). Compare also Novak (ed.) 1982.

18. Dennis 1993, p. xii. Against this must now be set the contention in Wilkinson 1996 (p. 166) that "when you compare children of lone parents with equally poor children brought up by both parents, most of the differences disappear." But until this dissident conclusion is shown to have survived critical examination I have no reason to reject the previous consensus.
19. Dennis and Erdos 1992, p. 26. They add in note 16 that "We would be very grateful to have our attention drawn to any study that contradicts what...must be seen as an astonishingly bold remark." I have myself drawn the attention of Dennis to Wilkinson 1996 and have thus discovered that, as I suspected, Wilkinson's conclusions on this particular matter are not supported by any compelling research evidence.
20. All the above figures are drawn from tables in Morgan, Patricia, 1995, p. 156.
21. Ibid., p.157.
22. It should be noted much more often than it is that neither the increased availability of contraception nor the effort devoted to sex education in schools appears to have any discernable effect upon the statistics of births outside marriage—or, for that matter, on those of teenage pregnancies terminated by abortion. See, for instance, White, Margaret, 1994, *Children and Contraception—Time to Change?* See also her 1999 *The Safe Sex Hoax!* Anyone reading *Teenage Pregnancy*, the Report from the Social Exclusion Unit Published by Her Majesty's Stationery Office in June 1999, should be aware of the devastating criticism of it published by, among many other individuals and organizations, the Campaign for Real Education.
23. Himmelfarb 1995, p. 253.
24. For discussion of the form of feminism that is so influential in and through such organizations, see Quest, Caroline (ed.), 1994, *Liberating Women...From Modern Feminism.*
25. Morgan 1995, chapter 2.
26. Ibid., quoted on p. 20.
27. Giddens 1998, p. 91.
28. Ibid., p. 89.
29. Ibid., p. 89.
30. Ibid., p. 90.
31. Ibid., p. 92.
32. Dennis and Erdos 1992, p. 20.
33. Abundant evidence about this campaign can be found in this work: e.g. pp. viii, 2, 24, 30-1, 44-5, 58, 88, 90, and 92.
34. This analogy is developed by Michael Levin in Caroline Quest (ed.) 1992, pp. 72-86.
35. Norman Barry discusses the changes needed in Caroline Quest (ed.) 1992, pp. 38-58.
36. Quoted in Morgan 1995, p. 97.
37. Malinowski, Bronislaw, 1927, p. 213 (emphasis added).

4

Self-Improvement and Social Action

Heaven helps those who help themselves is a well-tried maxim embodying in a small compass the results of vast human experience. The spirit of self-help is the root of all genuine growth in the individual; and, exhibited in the lives of many, it constitutes the true source of national vigour and strength. Help from without is often enfeebling in its effects, but help from within invariably invigorates. Whatever is done for *men or classes, to a certain extent takes away the stimulus and necessity of doing for themselves; and when men are subjected to over-guidance and over-government, the inevitable tendency is to render them comparatively helpless.*
—Samuel Smiles, Self-Help with Illustrations of Conduct and Perseverance *(1859)*

There are two very different ways in which we may hope to make the world better. One is through collective action, which in our time is usually the action of the central or the local state. The other is through the spontaneous improvement of ourselves and others as individuals. Both of these approaches are essential, they do not have to be mutually exclusive, and they can often be usefully complementary. But on particular occasions and for tackling particular problems one can be more relevant, more appropriate, and more productive than the other.

It was for a long time, and in some circles still is, a social policy orthodoxy to treat poverty, unemployment, ill health, and other conditions giving rise to entitlements of the receipt of welfare state benefits as if these conditions were afflictions falling always and only upon completely passive victims. But that, of course, is simply not the case. For some, at least some of these conditions come about, at least in part, because of the way that those subject to them and/or their associates have chosen to act. These conditions have not, that is to say, been inevitable.

Several of the major life-threatening or disabling diseases, notably, for instance, heart disease, respiratory diseases, and AIDS, are related to the kind of life their victims chose to lead—whether they smoked, what they ate, or the nature and extent of their sexual activities. Even poverty is now increasingly linked not with inevitable old age but with the disruption of, or the failure to form, families. Yet single parenthood and divorce both result from the choices of individuals.

The crucial part played by the choices of individuals in what are seen as "social" problems becomes manifest whenever two persons or two families become subject to the same conditions of unemployment, the same drug temptations, or the same inner city deprivation, and one makes the right choices while the other does not. Precisely because this chosen element is one of the individual's own choosing it is outside the direct control of government. No amount of tax-funded state spending can affect this wayward element directly.

It is not, however, beyond influence. The choices of individuals are affected by incentives. Government should surely be asking itself more often than it does whether current blanket health provision and current blanket relief for poverty do not encourage unhealthy and socially destructive choices. Even more importantly, government and others with influence should lose no opportunity of insisting upon the individual responsibility that necessarily accompanies the making of choices.

Signs of Collectivist and Statist Times

It was, however, a sign of our times that throughout her premiership of the United Kingdom (1979-1991), Margaret Thatcher was forever provoking choruses of condemnation by insisting that, although many of the things that can and ought to be done can only be done by government or by some other collective, there is also a good deal that individuals as individuals both can do and ought to do, both to better themselves and (immediately or ultimately) to benefit other people. It is perhaps even more significant of the extent of the contemporary popular preference for social over individual reform that clerical voices were among the loudest in their condemnation of that insistence. For some still living can remember when Christians typically insisted that we are members of a kind of creatures who can and cannot but make choices, that just this is the ground for human pretensions to a peculiar dignity, and that we alone are ultimately responsible for the senses in which we make whatever choices may from time to time be open to us. (On occasions, in those days, there was even some talk of a future life with perhaps hints on how for every individual the quality of that life would supposedly be determined by the senses of his or her most important choices on this earth).

Nowadays, however, expectations of ecclesiastical sympathy and support for such "individualism" must often be disappointed. Certainly some churches, and many members of all the others, maintain a commitment to individual conversion with consequent transformations in the lives of converts. Those North American churches, for instance, whose missionaries have in Guatemala and other countries of Latin America been making wholesale conversions to a traditional kind of Protestantism, have thereby produced transformations in individual lives, and consequently in entire communities, which are reminiscent of the original impact in the eighteenth- and early nineteenth-century England and Wales of John Wesley and his Methodist preachers.[1]

A few years after Margaret Thatcher entered office, Digby Anderson, a cleric who is also director of the Social Affairs Unit, brought together the team which, under his editorship, produced *The Kindness that Kills: The Churches' Simplistic Response to Social Issues*. His Introduction summed up their findings from studies of twenty-four then-recent pronouncements issued in the name of various church organizations or organizations of churches in the United Kingdom:

> Bluntly, if the Churches are to comment on specific and controversial socio-economic issues, they should work harder at being informed and scrupulously even-handed. Their publications are variously found to be sloppy, ill-thought out, ignorant, one-sided, addicted to secular fashions, uncritical of conventional "progressive" wisdom, hysterical, unmethodical in their uses of sources and evidence, theologically desiccated and, most deplorable, uncharitable to those who disagree.[2]

In that otherwise fairly comprehensive condemnation Digby Anderson neglected one of the most remarkable features common to almost all of these documents. For typically they had emphasized needs for and possibilities of collective action, and usually action by some level of government, rather than, and even to the complete exclusion of, any needs for or possibilities of actions by individuals to benefit both themselves and others.

What was truly most remarkable about this emphasis was that it should have been coming from groups of people claiming to be *speaking as Christians*. For traditionally Christian churches have of course been above all concerned with the salvation of individual human beings, and with collectives only and precisely in so far as these essentially consist of nothing else but their individual members. So it becomes indeed a remarkable indication of the strength, nature, and pervasiveness of the spirit of our times that those who speak on behalf of Christian churches should, in addressing social problems, write in a way scarcely distinguishable from that now so characteristic of most of their secular contemporaries.

It is perhaps just worth noting here, as an aside, that the remark made by Margaret Thatcher during her prime ministership for which she was most abused then, and for which she still—and not only in the UK—continues occasionally to be abused in her retirement, was a remark to the effect that human collectives "consist of nothing else but their individual members." What she actually said, in an interview printed in *Woman's Own* for October 31, 1987, was: "I don't believe in Society. There is no such thing, only individual people, and there are families." A delightful way of embarrassing Marxists who abused Margaret Thatcher on this account was to quote from *The Holy Family*, an early work by Karl Marx and Friedrich Engels:

> History does *nothing*; it "does *not* possess immense riches" it "does *not* fight battles." It is *men*, real living men, who do all this, who possess things and fight battles. It is not "history" which uses men as a means of achieving—as if it *were* an individual person—*its own* ends. History is nothing but the activity of men in pursuit of their ends (emphases original).

About eighteen months after the publication of *The Kindness that Kills*, which is a similar period before the making by Margaret Thatcher of that much abused remark, the Archbishop of Canterbury's Commission on Urban Priority Areas (UPA's) produced *Faith in the City: A Call for Action by Church and Nation.*[3] This was, of course, though bulky, only one document; it spoke directly for only one of the mainstream, still professedly Christian churches. But, although *Faith in the City* was only one document, it came as a climax to a series, and it served as the inspirational prelude to much subsequent action and publication. Though it spoke directly for only one particular organization, much of the same ideas, assumptions, and attitudes were to be found in statement after statement coming from most of the other affiliates of the British Council of Churches.

Nor is *Faith in the City* to be dismissed as having expressed only the opinions of fifteen Archiepiscopal Commissioners, however carefully handpicked. For it was later endorsed and adopted, apparently without significant reservations, by the Synod—the nearest thing to a Governing Body possessed by the Church of England. Again, although that organization manifestly is, and for many years past has been, in more than one sense, in secular decline it still remains, at least in England, "the church by law established."

On beginning to examine this *Call for Action by Church and Nation* it soon becomes clear that it is a call for government to make and for citizens to support government in making substantial all-round increases in tax-financed expenditure on state-supplied health, education, and welfare services. Certainly there is a paragraph that begins by conceding that "Individual responsibility and self-reliance are excellent objectives. The nation cannot do without them."[4] But, having seized every previous opportunity earlier in the Report not to stress or even to mention either their importance or their excellence, the Commissioners proceeded to italicize their own conviction, sustained by absolutely no deployment of evidence or argument, "*that at present too much emphasis is being given to individualism, and not enough to collective obligation.*"[5]

Again, it is clear that the Commissioners had at least heard tell of *The Kindness that Kills*. Nevertheless, we find, on a careful reading, that at no point did they allow themselves to be influenced either by it or by anything else originating from sources similarly suspect to all "progressive" persons. For the nearest that they ever came to citing those, or any other, infamous dissidents was in a dismissive aside: "the original provision of sewerage and piped water in our cities could clearly not be called a 'Kindness that Kills.'"[6] Indeed it could not; and, of course, by the authors of *The Kindness that Kills,* it never was.

In that public health context the Commissioner's contemptuous response to critics was peculiarly outrageous. For their Report nowhere made the slightest attempt to show, what in fact was and still remains the opposite of the truth, that the major problems and possibilities today still are—as at the time, over a century ago, of "the original provision of sewerage and piped water," they truly were—problems that can only be solved and possibilities that can only be realized by state action.

The Moralist's Temptation

While thus refusing to put that heavy emphasis upon individual responsibility which was, and in some places such as rural Guatemala still is, the glory of Protestant Christianity, the Commissioners nevertheless undeviatingly and systematically succumbed to what might be dubbed the Moralist's Temptation. This is the temptation to judge public policies as one might quite properly judge individual agents: by reference, that is, not so much to the actual effects of those policies as to the presumed intentions of their promoters. What, therefore, we lose on the roundabouts, we also lose on the swings.

Both faults can be found in the treatment of education: the first in the failure to say anything about truancy, the rates of which are certainly far higher in poor urban areas than elsewhere. Since knowledge and skills are not substances that can be poured into passive pots it is not sufficient to provide varied and abundant teaching, however excellent in quality. It is necessary also to have pupils willing and able to expose themselves to and to cooperate with that teaching. So it should be obvious that ensuring the exposure and cooperation is a very important thing that individual parents and their individual children both could do and ought to do both to better themselves and, immediately or ultimately, to benefit other people. It is also very much to the present point to add that, if only more children and more parents would in this respect now do what they could do and ought to do, then one most desirable effect would be that many children would eventually become more employable than would otherwise be the case, and hence less likely to be numbered among the future unemployed.

The second fault is shown in the Commission's assumptions: that, under the British or any similar system for the tax-funded state monopoly provision of primary and secondary educational services, you can be assured of getting the amount of pupil learning the taxpayers are paying for; and that any substantial improvements can and will be obtained only by a comparably substantial input of additional resources. These are assumptions which, understandably enough, all the supply side interest groups are concerned to promote. Yet they are also accepted much more widely, and this despite an ever more abundant accumulation of falsifying evidence.

At the time when the Commissioners were composing their Report, precise and reliable truancy statistics, taking account of actual unlicensed absence after the morning register had been taken, were not available. The Ministry responsible, then known as the Department of Education and Science (DES), did not encourage investigation of Post Registration Truancy (PRT), presumably anxious lest the findings of such research should be recognized as casting some discredit upon its stewardship.

The first direct, systematic, and officially funded research on PRT was completed only in 1989.[7] But none of its findings should have been much of a surprise to anyone who had noticed those of a survey taken by the Institute of Mathematics in 1977.[8] In this the same studiously elementary test was given to 8,000 pupils in state-maintained secondary schools in England and Wales. All the pupils tested were eligible to cease their schooling during the subsequent year, although the sample included its quota of those intending to continue their education voluntarily. There were large variations as between different Local Education Authorities (LEAs). These correspond, roughly, to school boards in the USA. The schools in which these tests were given were schools subject to, and had been selected as representative by, six very different LEAs up and down the country.

As usual the most deplorable levels of performance were achieved under the since-dissolved Inner London Education Authority (ILEA), an authority which—as the Commissioners should have noticed, but apparently did not—was contriving to spend more per pupil than any other, and 40 to 50 percent more than the national average.[9]

For instance, of London's sixteen-year-olds 25 percent were unable to multiply 6 by 79 even with a pencil and paper. The Institute concluded, with restraint, that "None of the results…for any authority is satisfactory. They all give strong support to the concern that has been expressed for some years and in many quarters about the level of numeracy among school leavers."

Furthermore, this survey by the Institute of Mathematics—published seven years before *Faith in the City*—produced by serendipity a most unsought finding, namely Post Registration Truancy (PRT). For actual post-registration absenteeism was everywhere higher than that officially registered and returned—rising under ILEA to 25 percent.

In the whole chapter "Education and Young People" there is little recognition of any defects in the supply of educational services which would not be simply remedied by massive shots of taxpayers' money. After noting that the new GCSE examinations were supposedly "designed for only 60 percent of the year group" and that "in some UPA schools" this would in fact disqualify considerably more than

40 percent of the pupils, the Commissioners proceeded to proffer a prime specimen of that uncritical acceptance of conventional "progressive" wisdom against which the authors of *The Kindness that Kills* so ruefully and, it appears, so ineffectually protested.

The Commission's one positive educational suggestion constituted a paradigm case of addiction to "secular fashions" and of being "uncritical of conventional 'progressive' wisdom." For, after noting that the then-new General Certificate of Secondary Education (GCSE) examinations were supposedly "designed for only 60 percent of the year group," and that "in some UP schools" this must disqualify considerably more than 40 percent of the pupils, they concluded, "The need in such schools is for a curriculum and an assessment system which affirms success rather than records failure."[10]

The actual need, nationally and not only "in some UPA schools," was at that time a comprehensive system of independently assessed leaving examinations. This would have provided a certification of employability, guaranteeing at least a minimum literacy and a minimum numeracy, as well perhaps as embracing whatever other useful skills particular pupils had contrived to acquire. For at the time when *Faith in the City* was published, up to half of those leaving ILEA schools at the first legal opportunity were leaving with no such independent evidence showing how if at all they had benefited from their years of compulsory schooling.

One rarely noticed consequence of that deficiency was that official committees established to make recommendations about illiteracy or innumeracy had to begin their deliberations by scratching around for evidence of the extent of the problems. The flip side of the same deficiency was that there was at that time no means of determining the total output of that huge and exceptionally important industry. But of course many critics reasonably recognized that very fact as the strongest of those various evidencing reasons that were publicly available for suspecting that it was indeed in appalling shape. These suspicions were quite dramatically confirmed by Sir Keith Joseph, who had served as a much-frustrated minister of state at the DES throughout the four years of the 1983-7 Thatcher administration. For after his retirement from that office and consequent elevation to the House of Lords, he described the condition of the entire UK state-maintained educational system in a debate about a long-awaited Education Reform Bill as constituting "a national catastrophe."[11]

Anyone puzzled by the Commissioners' desire for an examination system that "affirms success rather than records failure" should compare this recommendation with that on what they delicately described as "the arrival in our cities of large numbers of adherents to other faiths." It was that clergy should not be laggard in "affirming other cultures."[12] In both cases these recommendations clearly sprang from a reluctance to face awkward facts. In the case of the former it was the awkward fact of academic non-achievement that had to be concealed.[13] In the case of the latter what was meant by "affirming" was "adopting a positive attitude towards," but without on any account pressing awkward questions as to whether one culture is better adapted to some environments than another[14] or whether the faith of one culture is nearer the truth than that of any other. For these Commissioners were, as should have been noted much more widely than it was, remarkably reluctant to insist upon the truth of propositions traditionally rated essential to the religious faith in the name of which they were laboring to promote their preferred political prescriptions.

Statistics of absences from school must certainly not be construed as viable indices of truancy. For many of the absentees will have had some acceptable excuse. But PRT by definition just is truancy. And truancy is relevant to us because attending school and trying to learn is something individuals as individuals both can do and ought to do, both to better themselves and (immediately or ultimately) to benefit other people. This was, presumably, at least part of the reason why the Archbishop's Commissioners—being, as they obviously were, "addicted to secular fashions"—had nothing to say about truancy and hence about what both the truanting children themselves and their parents could do and ought to do to increase educational achievement. It is also very much to the general point to add that, if those children and their parents would do these things then one most important and desirable result should be that the children would become more employable and hence less likely to be numbered among the future unemployed.

Health and "Social" Justice

Health is another of the areas in which there is a great deal that individuals as individuals both can and ought to do, both to better themselves and (immediately or ultimately) to benefit other people, even though in a country with a National Health Service, there is no doubt that much can be achieved only through central government action. Guided by the "Black Report," the Archbishop's Commissioners were interested primarily in its subject, *Inequalities in Health*.[15] Characteristically they gave no consideration whatsoever to any possibilities of self-improvement. Also, here, as everywhere, they worked on the fashionable, false assumption that justice—or, at any rate, justice with the unexplained qualification "social"—is to be identified with (a no doubt somehow limited) equality of outcome. This perhaps explains the dogmatic yet surely misguided confidence of the motto of their chapter 8: "It is not charity when the powerful help the poor...it is justice."[16]

If and so far as the concern with such inequalities is a concern to raise the lowest levels so that they equal the highest rather than to achieve equality regardless—a protasis which is by no means always satisfied—then it becomes imperative to take on board the truth "that our life style may have more of an impact on our dying from certain diseases than all the most modern techniques of medical care." Consider, for instance, one extreme inequality revealed by the U.S. medical statistics. The adjacent states of Utah and Nevada are very similar in most respects—income levels, the availability of medical services, and so on. Yet, "Adult death rates for Nevada are *generally* 40 to 50 percent higher than for Utah. Death rates from cirrhosis of the liver and lung cancer among males in their thirties are almost *seven* times as high in Nevada as in Utah."[17]

It would appear that there was one debatable issue, and perhaps only one, upon which Nancy Reagan, her husband, and Jesse Jackson were in unqualified and uncompromising agreement. For they were forever, albeit all to little effect, advising youngsters, and everyone else tempted to take narcotics, "Just say 'No!'" The same unfashionable and widely unwelcome prescription clearly constituted and still remains the sovereign prophylactic against some other hugely damaging indulgences.

Thus, in his report *On the State of the Public Health for the Year 1987*,[18] the chief medical officer of Her Majesty's Government categorically asserted that smoking, though the habit was slowly declining, remained "the single most preventable cause of death and sickness." Noting that more girls than boys are now acquiring the habit, he added "that smoking in pregnancy is one of the most important known unfavourable factors affecting the health of the infant in the perinatal period." Excessive drinking, on the other hand, seemed to be on the increase. These indulgences, therefore, "represent a tragic waste of human resources, which also imposes a heavy burden on the health service."

Such information might well lead British non-smokers who are either moderate drinkers or teetotalers to wonder why they (we!) should be forced to bear the costs of countering the health effects of other people's over-indulgences—an inequity that could surely be remedied by introducing a system of (partial) insurance instead of the present (total) tax-funding of the National Health Service. In the nineteenth century, when little was known about either tobacco or alcohol as direct dangers to health, the recognized ill consequences of over-indulgence in alcohol were primarily the neglect and maltreatment of children by their besotted parents, and the battering and financial deprivation of wives by drunken husbands. Then the immediate reaction of most of the people who, rightly, perceived such evils to be a major social problem—and especially of "the people called Methodists"[19]—was: first, to set a personal example by signing the pledge of total abstinence; and thereafter, to labor to persuade others to sign and to keep that pledge.

The situation was already very different during the Thatcher administrations. When a junior government minister in one of them was so tactless as to point out that a great deal (but certainly not all) of the differences between the health statistics of different regions of the UK can be explained in terms of differences in the relative prevalence in those regions of various healthy and unhealthy habits, clerics were as eager as all other left-minded persons to join in the chorus of condemnation. They too insisted that these differences were inequalities; as such (socially) unjust; and hence to be rectified simply and solely by further infusions of tax-funded health care resources into the regions with worse than average health statistics.

Deplorable though it is that anyone should suffer lung cancer, it is, surely, precisely not *unjust* that any actual sufferers should have been heavy smokers rather than non-smokers. If and in so far as there is any wrongdoing here that is specifically *unjust*, it must lie in any injuries that might be done by smokers to other people. If, for instance, it were to be proved that passive smoking could result in lung cancer, which by the time of writing it certainly had not been, then active smokers would be guilty of injuring, and thus doing a without prefix or suffix injustice to (some of) those forced to breathe their smoke.[20]

These truths about the extent of ultimately self-inflicted ill health and the often-lamentable effects upon other people of choices endangering one's own health cannot honestly be avoided or evaded, as so many would wish to do, by pointing to positive correlations between socio-economic class membership and certain of the relevant dangerous indulgences. *The Nation's Health: A Strategy for the 1990s*, by Alwyn Smith and B. Jacobson, was very much in the tradition of *Inequalities in Health*, the earlier report which served as a prime source for the relevant chapter of *Faith in the City*. Indeed, one of its members was a secular adviser to the Archbishop's Commission.

The Times reported both his, Professor David Donnison's, and Professor Alwyn Smith's comments on the day after publication.[21] Once again they emphasized the extent to which ill health can be the result of forces such as income variation over which individuals have little or no control. As so often, a correlation between income variation and mortality rates was assumed to indicate direct cause. The government was blamed for somehow "encouraging" the greater inequalities that allegedly caused ill health. This same argument is frequently used to suggest that increasing subsidies to the poor and correspondingly increasing taxation of others will do more for health than would curative medicine, and indeed this particular Report's authors stressed that government policy must provide the solution for all health problems. But correlations are not reliable indices of direct causal connections. Nor does everything that may properly be called a direct cause deterministically necessitate.

Two other things need to be said immediately about the assumption that all patients—or, at any rate, all those who are members of those groups said to need either further handouts of other people's money and/or new government policies—are helpless creatures of their "socio-economic circumstances" rather than responsible (or, sometimes, very irresponsible) agents, who could and often do fall "into the hands of the health professions" as a result of something they themselves avoidably did or failed to do.

First, this assumption appears not to be consistent with the claim, such as that made in the following paragraph of the report in *The*

Times, that there have been significant improvements "in three areas...AIDS, alcohol and illegal drug misuse..." Second, that self-same tactless junior minister once again pitched in by objecting that to assume such necessitating determinism is, as indeed it is, insulting: "That really does patronise people. Everybody has the right and some opportunity to improve their own health."

Low Pay or no Pay?

Similar patronizing assumptions are extremely widespread among those who, like David Sheppard the Bishop of Liverpool and one of the Archbishop's Commissioners, advocate a *Bias to the Poor*.[22] They are, for instance, implicit in the very name of the Low Pay Unit, thanked by the Archbishop's Commissioners for submitted written evidence. This self-description suggests that the problem is conceived as one of somehow raising the rates of pay for all those sorts of jobs that are at present accounted low paid. If that is indeed the problem, then the solution is bound to be collectivist, presumably involving the introduction of minimum wage laws or some equivalent thereto.

There are, however, three very serious objections to the policies thus prejudicially endorsed. First, almost everyone who has ever sincerely sought to discover the actual consequences of introducing minimum wage laws seems to have concluded that they increase unemployment. Yet, surely, low pay is better than no pay?[23]

Second, low paid jobs, even if not, as they often are, the first steps on a formalized career ladder, can be made, and by many people have been and are being made, the first stages in their own individual advancement. In the USA before World War II those lacking special skills could often, by pricing themselves into unskilled jobs, make themselves more employable by acquiring the basic good habits of timekeeping and application. Minimum wage laws make this sort of self-help impossible. One clear consequence—despite the intervening explosion of civil rights legislation—has been that, whereas in the thirties the rates of black juvenile unemployment were lower than those for whites, the reverse is now the case.[24]

Third, a great many of the jobs that are accounted low paid are in fact providing some household with its second or even third income; an income which, as an additional income, may well be making all the difference between modest prosperity and genuine hardship-causing poverty. In so far as this is the case a job-destroying rise in the minimum wage is likely to diminish the perceived scandal of low pay only at the paradoxical cost of increasing the number of households in actual poverty.

These three considerations weighed heavily with Michael Novak and his colleagues at the Working Seminar on Family and American Welfare Policy when they made their report. They concluded (writing in the middle eighties) that in the USA:

> The probabilities of remaining involuntarily in poverty are remarkably low for those who, first, complete high school, then, once adult, get and stay married (even if not for the first try), and, finally, stay employed, even at a wage and under conditions below their ultimate aims.[25]

There were two emphases in all the work done by Michael Novak's Seminar that British readers may find unfamiliar, and perhaps refreshing. This first is upon the family and, above all the intact family, as both potentially and actually by far the most important of all institutions promoting health, education, and welfare. The second is upon the even more obvious fact that families are formed (or not formed) as the result of the congruent choices of two people, one male and one female, and that, when standard families degenerate into the one-parent variant form, this too now almost always results from a choice made by at least one of the parents, usually the male. (The exception, in these days happily rare, is when one becomes a widow or a widower).[26]

Once upon a time it could reasonably have been assumed that any statement on social policy made on behalf of a church with pretensions to Christian catholicity would have emphasized these two rather obvious truths. But this, it appears, is true no longer. For when the authors of *Faith in the City* wrote about marriage and families at all,[27] they wrote of the failure to form families, and of the disruption of formed families into one-parent families, as if these were occurrences beyond human control. In such natural disasters as typhoons and hurricanes there is indeed nothing anyone can do—save try to limit the damage and help the inevitable victims. But this is different. Certainly there are victims needing help—mainly the children. But there are victimizers as well as victims. And these victimizers are—like us and like their victims—agents, who therefore in principle can, and in practice surely should, be held responsible for whatever they have done or failed to do.

The chapter "Church and City" rated the "incidence of marriage and other family problems," both nationally and still more in the UPAs, as significantly albeit not vastly more serious than "level of unemployment" or "quality/price of public transport" or "number of elderly people."[28] Yet, it still seemed never to occur to the Archbishop's Commissioners that these top-rated marriage and other family problems might themselves be prime causes of some of the others. Significantly too they chose to speak of "marriage breakdown," as if the failure to form marriages or their disruption was itself beyond human control.

No one pretending to have studied or to have attempted solving such problems has any business to be unaware of the evidence that the absence of a concerned father makes it much more likely that the children thus deprived will under-achieve educationally and/or become delinquent.[29] Asserting that blacks were disproportionately represented not only among the unemployed but also among educational underachievers and the prison population, the unevidenced knee-jerk reaction of the Archbishop's Commissioners was to put this down to racism—although they did somewhat prissily allow that a lot of unemployed black youths "had fathers...living away from home."[30]

By sometimes (but not consistently) following the obscurantist usage under which all non-whites are brigaded together as blacks, *Faith in the City* concealed both the size and the likely prime cause of the differences between the track records of British Afro-Caribbeans and British Asians. But researchers for ILEA, which was in the forefront of campaigns to encourage all non-whites to see themselves as chronically victimized by and outcast from white British society, continued to come up with statistics discrediting their employer's presuppositions. These statistics showed that, although there were—as should be expected—substantial performance differences between different subsets of these racial sets, the Asians in general were doing much better than the whites and the blacks, or at least than those blacks whose parents or grandparents came from the Caribbean. For the statistics showed that, whereas 20 percent of all the children in these schools came from one-parent families, this was true of 43 percent of the Afro-Caribbeans but only of 5 percent of the Asians.[31]

For such social problems the sovereign remedy is not the comfortably remote social action of "affirming other cultures," as recommended by *Faith in the City*,[32] but the costly and laborious individual actions of parents of both sexes and all races to fulfill their own parental responsibilities. (The choice of the word "affirm" was a characteristically evasive compromise between courageously continuing to assert the truth of the Christian revelation and outright conceding to the militants of multiculturalism that all cultures, with perhaps the exception of our own, are equally good or equally "valid").

What Faith in the City?

When *Faith in the City* was first published, it was said in the general press that some Conservative Members of Parliament, none of whom were ever, so far as I know, actually named, had attacked it as a Marxist document. That it certainly was not. But at that time there certainly was one most important professedly Christian organization that could truly be accused, if not of producing Marxist documents, of supporting Marxist causes. That was the World Council of Churches (WCC). Most Protestant churches, including the Church of England, were, and still are, affiliated to it.

In pursuing its programs for "combating racism" and "promoting liberation," the WCC in the seventies and early eighties funded and in other ways supported various organizations of revolutionary "freedom fighters" battling to establish Communist or Communist-type regimes. Thus, while continuing to support the pro-Soviet Sandinistas against the Contras in Nicaragua, the WCC also supported another band of Communist-type "freedom fighters" struggling to overthrow a Christian Democratic government in Honduras! Perhaps most scandalous of all was the WCC's support, including funding, for ZANU-PF, the association of "freedom fighters" under Robert Mugabe, the future president of the future Zimbabwe. For ZANU-PF, during its "liberation" struggles, murdered white missionaries along with many of their black converts, and this without provoking any audible protest from the WCC. Nor was the WCC ever heard to protest the persecution of Christians in the USSR or in any of its satellites.[33]

The only explicit references to Marx or Marxism in *Faith in the City* are to be found at the beginning of a paragraph under the heading "The Tradition of Christian Social Thought." The relevant sentences are:

It is against the background of the excessive individualism of much Christian thinking in the nineteenth century that we must place Marx's perception that evil is to be found, not just in the human heart, but in the very structures of economic and social relationships. This perception is also found to a notable degree in the Old Testament (from which, in fact, Marx may have derived it), where there is explicit recognition of the inevitable tendency of the rich to get richer and the poor to get poorer unless some constraint is imposed to limit the freedom of individuals to profit without restraint from a market economy. Most ancient societies were aware of this tendency. But the Old Testament is unique in attempting to impose a number of controls upon society to check the inevitable increase of social and economic inequalities.

We must here suspect that, had we been able to refer to the passages the Commissioners had in mind, we should have found that they contained references only to poverty but not to inequalities.[34] What it is here suggested that Marx might have derived from the Old Testament was what is normally called the Immiseration Thesis. This, in its first formulation, in the *Communist Manifesto*, read: "The modern labourer, instead of rising with the progress of industry, sinks deeper and deeper below the conditions of existence of his own class."[35] That was for Marx a thesis that applied to a capitalist industrial system as opposed to a purely agricultural economy and which would, he contended, inevitably result in the decisive overthrow of that capitalist system by a proletarian revolution. By the time that he published *Capital*, the great work that was going to prove this essential thesis, Marx knew that actually it was false. He dealt with this theoretical difficulty by simply omitting from *Capital* all reference to this decisive falsifying evidence.[36]

But now, given that the Immiseration Thesis is false, at least as applied to capitalist countries, what are we to say about this supposedly "inevitable tendency of the rich *to get richer and the poor to get poorer* unless some constraint is imposed to limit the freedom of individuals to profit without restraint from a market economy" (emphasis now added)? One possible move is the argument that, at least in a primitive, entirely agricultural economy it was possible, even likely, that the poor would become progressively poorer if bad years left them with debts that they could not pay off in subsequent good years. Although obviously, this is not relevant to the economy with which the Archbishop's Commissioners were concerned, it may perhaps be of interest to note that the Pentateuch makes provision for dealing with the problem.[37] Thus, various portions of the harvest were set aside for the poor—the corner of the field, the forgotten sheaf, and so on (*Leviticus*, 19:9-10; *Deuteronomy*, 24:19-21). On the third and sixth years of the seven-year cycle, they were given a tenth of all produce (*Deuteronomy*, 26:12). And in the seventh year, all outstanding debts were remitted (*Deuteronomy*, 15:1-2). This last provision was clearly open to circumvention. So there is another provision against that:

> Be careful that you do not have a base thought and say to yourself "The seventh year is approaching, and it will be the remission year." You may look unkindly on your impoverished brother, and not give him anything. If he then complains to God about you, you will be guilty of sin (*Deuteronomy*, 15:9).

Another possible move is implicitly to define the extremes of poverty and riches in terms of the inequality that subsists between them. This is the move made by the inventors of permanent poverty.[38] For anyone who wanted to continue to recognize envy as a deadly sin this would be an awkward line to take. But apparently it did not embarrass those who, many years ago, issued on behalf of the Labour Party a pamphlet entitled simply *Equality* and colored green. A second possible move, falsely assumed to be not merely consistent with but actually required by old-fashioned without prefix or suffix justice, rules that everyone's condition must be made as close as practicable to that of everyone else. This second move will be discussed in chapter 5, below.

Anyone who had ever read any church statements on political and social matters made in earlier periods must have been astonished to find so little attempt made by *Faith in the City* to show how its conclusions were, if not derived from, then at least guided by Christian beliefs. For instance, as has just been noticed, readers were not provided with references that would have enabled them to check claims about the Old Testament sources from which Marx might have derived the Immiseration Thesis.

Any initial suspicion that many of the Commissioners were not so much concerned to discover public policy implications in Gospel teaching as to rally the organizational and influential strength of the Church of England in support of their own antecedent political convictions—convictions that may have been as near as makes little matter, and totally secular in origin—is bound to be strengthened by the discovery that, in order to support all their political and social recommendations and to authenticate their own Christian credentials, they appeal to two and only two specific texts from the New Testament, and to none at all from any other traditional fount of

Christian authority. Both of these two appeals occur together on the same page.[39] Three words—"remember the poor"—are quoted as from *Galatians*, (ii) 10, and this particular injunction is backed up with a reference to *II Corinthians*, (vii)-(ix). There follows a mention of the Good Samaritan without—perhaps significantly—any reminder that that parable is to be found in *Luke*, (x) 30-5.

It should not be surprising that the Archbishop's Commissioners were able to offer so little in the way of New Testament authority for recommendations calling almost always for drastic measures from the state rather than for actions by individuals. What should have surprised us is their own general preference for state measures, and their own determination to ignore the possibilities of and the needs for individual action. That should have surprised us because, on traditional Christian assumptions, God chose to become incarnate long before anyone had every dreamed of the possibility of establishing a comprehensive, tax-financed, cradle-to-the-grave, welfare state. Yet it seems never to have occurred to the Commissioners that it must in consequence be an enormously difficult if not downright impossible task validly to derive much clear-cut political guidance for contemporary British voters from New Testament teachings. Instead they appear to have given no consideration at all to any possible objections before presenting, in the name of the Church of England, their confident call for substantial increases in tax-funded state spending on everything except the traditional and elementary functions of the state, namely, defense and the maintenance of law and order.

It was perhaps prudent of the Commissioners not to encourage close attention to the parable of the Good Samaritan. For he performed all the medical services needed by the robbed and injured traveller with his own hands, using his own materials. It was too from his own and not the taxpayers' purse that he afterwards undertook to pay for the victim's further accommodation: "And on the morrow when he departed, he took out two pence, and gave them to the host, and said unto him, 'Take care of him, and whatsoever thou spendest more, when I come again, I will repay thee.'" So it was to this parable that, a year or two after the first publication of *Faith in the City*, Margaret Thatcher referred in an address to the General Assembly of the Kirk of Scotland, which had associated itself with the policy recommendations of that work. Her critics then complained of the selectivity of this Biblical citation, apparently considering it some sort of fault to have chosen the most apt quotation to reveal the lack of Biblical support for their own demand for a substantial increase in tax-funded spending on the National Health Service!

Although the Archbishop's Commissioners showed a remarkable confidence in their political recommendations, and had apparently never felt any need to consider any contrary argument, they appear to have been somewhat less confident about their theology. "Philosophy," they tell us, "has moved far beyond Descartes and has finally exorcised 'the ghost in the machine': few philosophers now allow for a separate component, or 'soul'..."[40] Far be it from someone who was a graduate student supervised by Gilbert Ryle during the year in which he published *The Concept of Mind* to challenge that conclusion. But the Archbishop's Commissioners should have realized that it is one that threatens any doctrine of a future life.

It is simply not sufficient to say, as they do, that "Christian belief in life after death is properly expressed in terms of the Resurrection of the Body: the Greek conception of an immortal soul has never been able to give expression to it."[41] For it is only if and in as much as souls are conceived—as by Ryleans they most emphatically are not—as what philosophers call "substances" (namely, as things that can exist separately and, as it were, in their own right) that souls can significantly be said to first survive the deaths and dissolutions of the flesh-and-blood people whose souls they were, and later acquire resurrection bodies. In a Rylean view, to construe the assertion that someone has or really is a soul is like comparing the Red Queen's dog's loss of temper with the loss of his bone, or like looking for the grin remaining after the Cheshire cat itself has disappeared.[42]

The chapter in *Faith in the City* entitled "Theological Priorities" contained remarkably little about old-fashioned theology that had, "since the early centuries," as the Commissioners said, "been understood as a deductive science. Christian truth is conceived as a system, derived both from divine revelation and human reason, and growth in understanding is aided by historical and philosophical disciplines."[43] Although they allowed that "there can be no doubt of the value of critical study of the scriptures and of vigorous theological thinking," they nevertheless saw this as no longer in touch with the times and the life of the inner cities. So they hankered after "Liberation Theology" (always, unlike plain old-fashioned theology, given the reverent benefit of initial capital letters). This had, in Latin America,

> proposed a method and a set of priorities which reflect the concerns, not of the oppressors but of the oppressed, not of the rich but of the poor. In this context, theological reasoning has been relevant and in a certain sense "true" only if it results in a determination and a strategy to liberate the poor from this oppression.[44]

Apparently not embarrassed by any anxieties as to whether the conclusions of this new form of "theological reasoning" would be both, in a traditional understanding, genuinely theological and actually true as opposed to "in a certain sense 'true,'" the Commissioners went on to conclude that:

> To all of us, the example of Liberation Theology opens up the possibility that new priorities, as well as new methods, can restore us to a theology that is truly relevant to the needs and aspirations of people today.[45]

Britain's then Chief Rabbi was so disturbed by the teachings of *Faith in the City* that he took, for a Jewish leader, the unusual step of commenting unfavorably upon a professedly Christian document in a booklet entitled *From Doom to Hope*.[46] Christianity and Judaism, he wrote, both "raise the relief of want as a precept of the highest religious virtue." But against *Faith in the City* he objected that:

> ...whilst it distinguishes between work and unemployment...it falls short of hailing work as a virtue in itself...the Jewish work-ethic is rather more positive and demanding... Cheap labour is more dignified than a free dole, and industriousness generates greater wealth than increased wages for decreasing hours of work.

Whereas the authors of *Faith in the City* had insisted that "The creation of wealth must always go hand in hand with just distribution...there is a long Christian tradition, *reaching back to the Old Testament prophets*...which firmly rejects the amassing of wealth unless it is justly distributed,"[47] the then Chief Rabbi, whom we must assume to have been at least equally familiar with the prophetic books of the Old Testament, reminded them that:

> [W]hile Judaism obviously insists on unimpeachable rectitude in the acquisition of wealth and on the due allocation of a given percentage for charitable purposes...it never frowned on gaining wealth as such, nor demanded that wealth be shared or distributed to equalise rich and poor by some artificial balance, unrelated to effort and skill.

Cheap labor (Low Pay) is indeed more dignified than a free dole. So for Judaism the emphasis is always on both self-help and helping others to help themselves. The best of charity is that which helps the poor to dispense with charity and to escape dependency. It is, said Rabbi Moses ben Maimon (Maimonides to the Greeks)

> ...that of the person who assists the poor man by providing him with a gift or loan, or by accepting him into a business partnership, or by helping him find employment—in a word, by putting him where he can dispense with others people's aid.

Notes

1. See, for instance, Martin, David, *Tongues of Fire: The Explosion of Protestantism.*
2. Anderson (ed.) 1984, p. 2.
3. O'Brien, R. (Chairman), *Faith in the City: A Call for Action by Church and Nation* (London: Church House Publishing, 1980).
4. Ibid., p. 208.
5. Ibid., p. 208 (emphasis original).
6. Ibid., p. 212.
7. Aficionados of *Yes Minister* will appreciate the story of the junior minister who persisted in his efforts to get the first DES grant awarded to PRT researchers, and in consequence lost that ministerial position. See Flew, 1994, pp. 51-2.
8. The findings are most easily accessible, reprinted in Cox and Marks (eds.) 1982, pp. 59-66.
9. *Faith in the City* contains an Appendix F (pp. 389-397) "Written Evidence Received." The Commissioners' sole source of evidence about education would appear to have been ILEA itself! If the Commissioners had been prepared to admit the possibility that the state-maintained schools and, in particular those of ILEA, were not providing good value for money, they could have found plenty of evidence in Cox and Marks 1980 and Cox and Marks (eds.) 1982.
10. O'Brien (Chairman), 1985, p. 295.
11. *House of Lords Debates* for April 18, 1988, Column 1263. U.S. readers will naturally compare this statement with the comparably alarming verdict upon their own system in *A Nation at Risk.*
12. O'Brien (Chairman), 1985, p. 306.
13. See Phillips, Melanie, 1996, *All Must Have Prizes.*
14. Anyone wanting to achieve a real understanding of the relations of cultures should begin by studying Thomas Sowell 1981 (*Ethnic America*) and then proceed to Sowell 1994, 1996, and 1998.
15. London, Department of Health and Social Security, 1980. It is this that has come to be known as the "Black Report." Before anyone accepts this report as revealed truth they should first study Dr. James Le Fanu 1993.
16. O'Brien (Chairman), 1985, p. 169. For more on this curious and, surely, entirely unbiblical conception of justice, see chapter 5, below. The same David Sheppard, Bishop of Liverpool, who contributed this remarkable chapter motto, was reproached for the Biblical ignorance shown in the title of his book *Bias to the Poor* by a future chief rabbi. See note 22, below.
17. Both this and the subsequent similar quotation were drawn from Reading no. 25 in Lammers and Varhey 1987.
18. HM Chief Medical Officer, *On the State of the Public Health for the Year 1987* (London: Her Majesty's Stationery Office, 1988).

19. Once in a TV interview with Prime Minister Thatcher, Brian Walden spoke of Victorian values. He should surely have said, more specifically, Methodist. For Margaret Roberts was raised in a home above the family grocer's shop, and her admired father was a Methodist local preacher.
20. On this issue see, for instance, my "Passive Smoking, Scientific Method and Corrupted Sciences," in Schaler and Schaler (eds.) 1998.
21. September 23, 1988.
22. This title was attacked by Jonathan Sacks, the present Chief Rabbi, in his *Wealth and Poverty: A Jewish Analysis* (1985). On page 16 of this pamphlet he wrote: "The single point I might have made at the beginning but have chosen to leave to the end is that the one thing Judaism rules out *ab initio*, by specific Biblical command, is a bias to the poor. Precisely because its whole moral code is oriented towards compassion, the Bible uniquely found it necessary to command: 'You shall not favour a poor man in his cause' (*Exodus* 23:3, see *Leviticus* 19:15)."
23. See first "Minimum Wage, Maximum Folly," chapter 3 of Williams, Walter, 1982, and then proceed to his three later works.
24. See again Williams, Walter, 1982, loc. cit.
25. Novak (ed.) 1987, p. 5.
26. For a recent attempt to restore these two emphases compare Anderson and Dawson (eds.), 1986.
27. In other days such a volume would have included at least one whole chapter on these topics: not in 1985.
28. O'Brien (Chairman), 1985, pp. 39-40.
29. See, for instance, Morgan, Patricia, "Feminist Attempts to Sack Father: A Case of Unfair Dismissal?" in Anderson and Dawson (eds.), 1986.
30. O'Brien (Chairman), 1985, pp. 17, 302-3, and 327.
31. See my "Education against Racism" in O'Keeffe 1986 (ed.), and compare Palmer (ed.) 1986 passim.
32. O'Brien (Chairman), 1985, p. 306.
33. See Smith, Bernard, 1976 and Lefever, Ernest, 1979, and compare Tingle 1998.
34. I am not at this time in a position to check my memory of looking up the word "equal" in a concordance to the King James Bible and finding only two employments of the word "equal" and none for any of its derivatives.
35. Marx and Engels, 1968, p. 93.
36. This was, I believe, first pointed out in Wolfe, Bertram D., 1965, pp. 322-3.
37. The Pentateuchal material that follows was borrowed from page 6 of Sacks, Jonathan, 1985.
38. See Dennis, Norman, 1997, *The Invention of Permanent Poverty*.
39. O'Brien (Chairman), p. 47.
40. Ibid., p. 50.
41. Ibid., p. 51.
42. See Flew [1986] 2000, especially chapter 7.
43. O'Brien (Chairman), 1985, p. 63.
44. Ibid., pp. 63-4.
45. Ibid., p. 64. The best book, by a Roman Catholic, about Liberation Theology is Novak 1987.
46. All my information about the contents of this booklet was derived from Julius Gould's critical notice of *Faith in the City*, published in *Encounter* in 1986. Unfortunately, footnote 6, in which he presumably supplied the relevant publication data, was omitted in the printing.
47. O'Brien (Chairman), 1985, p. 53 (emphasis added).

5

Welfare Rights for the Formerly Disadvantaged

I want to be a man on the same basis and level as any white citizen—I want to be free as the whitest citizen. I want to exercise, and in full, the same rights as the white American. I want to be eligible for employment exclusively on the basis of my skills and employability, and for housing solely on my capacity to pay. I want to have the same privileges, the same treatment in public places as every other person...
—Dr. Ralph Bunche (the first black American to serve as, among many other things, U.S. Permanent Representative at the UN)

Chapter 2 expounded and criticized the doctrine of anti-social determinism, a doctrine tacitly presupposed by many of the workers in the welfare state machine and mistakenly believed to be implied by the findings of the human psychological and social sciences. Chapter 3 considered the way in which the existence of a welfare state, and the consequent entitlement of all its citizens to any and all of the welfare provisions it makes available, must tend to demoralize those citizens. Chapter 4 went on to point out implications of the observation that many of the unfortunate conditions for which welfare states provide relief are conditions into which many of their victims could by their own efforts have avoided falling in the first place and/or could sooner or later escape by their own efforts. It is now time to give further consideration to the problems produced by the establishment of welfare rights.

Welfare Rights as Opposed to Option Rights

The provisions of a welfare state are to be seen as goods of which all legitimate recipients have a welfare right. And whereas the rights proclaimed in the American Declaration of Independence were option rights—rights, that is to say, giving individuals freedom to choose between the various courses of action or inaction they perceive as being open to them—welfare rights are rights to receive some good. And whereas those option rights were clearly proclaimed as subsisting prior to the establishment of states, welfare rights implicitly presuppose the existence of states—and of comparatively prosperous states, at that—as the providers of welfare, the enjoyment of which is a right.

This point can be somewhat mischievously reinforced by referring to the Universal Declaration of Human Rights proclaimed over fifty years ago by the General Assembly of the United Nations. This 1948 Declaration was much longer[1] and much less well written than its American predecessor.[2] The rights it listed were in fact mainly welfare rights. Consider, for example, Article 25: "...everyone has the right to a standard of living adequate for the health and well-being of himself and of his family...and the right to security in the event of unemployment, sickness, disability, widowhood, old age or other lack of livelihood in circumstances beyond his control." Or, again, consider Article 26: "Everyone has the right to education. Education shall be free, at least in the elementary and fundamental stages. Elementary education shall be compulsory." And so, through a clause specifying that it must further the activities of the United Nations, on to the slightly incongruous afterthought conclusion that "parents have a prior right to choose the kind of education that shall be given to their children."

A New Kind of Welfare Rights

There were, long before 1948, arrangements in many countries for the state provision, available to all citizens as such, of various kinds of welfare services—primarily educational services of the kinds and quantities specified in this UN Declaration. And the entitlements of the citizens of those countries to those provisions can be seen as their welfare rights. What seems to have been invented first in the USA but has since been introduced in many other First World countries is, not simply a right to equal treatment as a citizen, but instead a right to equal treatment as a citizen who is also a member of some previously disadvantaged sub-category of citizens.

Legislation to establish welfare rights of this new kind—like legislation to impose rent controls and introduce environmental and planning regulations—has a very understandable appeal to members of elected legislatures. For it enables them to be seen to be doing good to (some of) their constituents but doing it without incurring general unpopularity by raising taxes in order to compensate the unfortunates thus forced to bear the costs of this beneficence.

The first set of U.S. citizens to be legally endowed with a welfare right to equal treatment as members of a category of the previously disadvantaged were blacks. Judged by the stated intentions of those who guided the 1964 Civil Rights Act through Congress, the introduction of that Act was a spectacular and immediate success. The barriers excluding blacks from public accommodation tumbled overnight, while all forms of open and systematic anti-black discrimination seem to have been effectively abolished soon after.

But this success did not satisfy either the unofficial civil rights movement or the bureaucracy set up to supervise the enforcement of the Civil Rights Act itself. The movement extended its ambitions beyond the elimination of merely negative discrimination against blacks and went on to demand more positive action in their favor,[3] while the activities of the Equal Employment Opportunities Commission (EEOC) have gone far to confirm the universal validity of Hastie's Law: "For all societies the amount of perceived racism varies directly with the number of those in that society whose pay and future career prospects depend upon the discovery of ever more racism to combat."[4] Hastie's Law thus constitutes a particular instance of the more comprehensive sociological law stating that when any substantial bureaucracy owes its existence to a perceived problem, that problem is never finally solved. Never ask the barber whether you need a haircut.

The other grounds of discrimination forbidden by the 1964 Act do not seem to have received much attention in any of the debates preceding its passage. But, once the general principle of legislating against particular grounds of discrimination in the making of hiring decisions had been accepted, age was quickly added to the list. Thus 1967 saw the passage of the Age Discrimination in Employment Act (ADEA). Since then other grounds have been added to the list in the USA and other countries have also introduced legislation to ban discrimination on various grounds. By so doing they have all criminalized discrimination against members of previously disadvantaged sub-categories of their citizens, and thus endowed members of these sub-categories with welfare rights of this new kind.

Because the Civil Rights Act 1964 was in the USA both so urgently necessary and so immediately successful in removing all forms of open and systematic discrimination against blacks, very little attention was then given to the implications of legislating against particular grounds of discrimination in hiring decisions. The other countries that, whether wittingly or unwittingly, have followed the U.S. example, by establishing such collective rights to non-discrimination, also seem to have followed the U.S. example of failing to investigate the fundamental implications for civil society and the economy of the establishment of such collective rights to non-discrimination. But they have failed with less excuse.

The key expression "civil rights" was originally used to refer to the civil capacity to contract, to own property, to make wills, to give evidence, and to sue and be sued. These are rights all individuals can enjoy simultaneously both against the state and against one another. Their accurate definition and faithful protection is indispensable for any regime of limited government and individual freedom, and for all persons regardless of race, creed, religion, sex, or national origin. But the development of what is now called civil rights legislation has progressively decreased the freedoms of all Americans to associate or to refuse to associate with whomsoever they may wish, and to make contracts upon whatever terms are mutually agreeable. In the name of diversity, the drive in the USA is towards an enforced uniformity of personnel distribution across all firms, and indeed, across all other associations and institutions.

This development was certainly not mandated by the 1964 Act. On the contrary: although much of what has since actually happened was foreseen by opponents, those steering the bill through the Senate insisted categorically and repeatedly, and in all sincerity and truth, that Title VII would prohibit rather than require quotas in the name of "racial balance" and various other outcomes feared by opponents. So critics of America's activist judges may find wry satisfaction in reacting, for instance, to statements made in a memorandum of reassurance provided by Senators Case and Clark, in their role as bipartisan captains for the Bill while it was being debated on the Senate floor, that:

> There is no requirement in title VII that an employer maintain a racial balance in his work force. On the contrary, any deliberate attempt to maintain a racial balance, whatever such a balance may be, would involve a violation of title VII because maintaining a balance would require an employer to hire or refuse to hire on the basis of race.

Similarly:

> Title VII would not require, *and no court could read Title VII as requiring*, an employer to lower or change occupational qualifications because proportionately fewer Negroes than whites are able to meet them (Quoted in Richard Epstein, 1992, p. 118; emphasis added).

Thanks, however, to "The imperatives of bureaucratic expansion and majoritarian politics...the Civil Rights Act" has, since it was originally passed, yielded in the USA a "massive, complex set of laws that has basically done two things: (1) made it permissible to discriminate at will against whites and men (especially white men), and (2) made it possible to charge race- or sex-neutral firms with discrimination on the strength of statistical techniques whose application is flawed at every crucial juncture" (Ibid., pp. 78-9).[5]

In terms of the crucial legal conceptions, the development has been from disparate treatment, which was what—and all that was—explicitly forbidden by the 1964 Act, to disparate impact, the very different offence that has since become effectively outlawed. Disparate treatment cases, "which involve efforts to show that the defendant's conduct was actuated by some illegitimate motive, often raise very delicate questions of procedure and proof, but these difficulties are of a sort with which the legal system can ordinarily cope, at least at a price" (Ibid., p. 160). Disparate impact cases are an altogether different matter. These impose "intolerable and unnecessary demands on both the legal system and affected employment markets." For they "allow courts to infer unlawful discrimination, wholly without evidence of improper motive, and solely from the (perceived) disparate consequences of certain hiring tests and procedures" (Ibid., p. 160).

Such was the success of the Civil Rights Act (1964) in effectively eliminating anti-black discrimination that it very soon became impossible to prepare prosecution cases that would stand up in court. But, in obedience to Hastie's Law, the EEOC refused to entertain the, for them, uncomfortable idea that the difficulty of proving that discrimination was still widespread might arise from the fact that, insofar as this could reasonably be expected in an always necessarily imperfect world, it had in fact ceased. Instead, with the assistance both of an ever activist judiciary and the pressures of the equally expansionist civil rights movement, the EEOC met its difficulty by introducing the radically different conception of disparate impact.

Since this was introduced as an element of somewhat complicated case law rather than by (indeed flatly against) a clear-cut Act of Congress, it may be helpful for us to approach by way of consideration the offence of indirect discrimination introduced by the UK Race Relations Act 1976. Direct discrimination is there defined as consisting in "treating a person, on racial grounds, less favourably than others would be treated in the same or similar circumstances." Indirect racial discrimination is a more complex concept, consisting in "applying a requirement or condition which, although applied equally to all racial groups, is such that a considerably smaller proportion of a particular racial group can comply with it and which cannot be shown to be justifiable on other than racial grounds."

Obviously, much must depend upon what is acceptable as an adequate justification "on other than racial grounds." But, quite apart from this, there are two most fundamental objections to the statutory introduction of the offence of indirect discrimination. The first of these was put by a future Lord Chancellor[6] in the original House of Commons debate: "It is a fundamental principle of English law, and one which is vital to the preservation of individual liberty, that a crime should consist of two elements: first there must be a prohibited act and then there should be a state of mind. Quite deliberately the Government have created in this new Clause an indictable offence in which the mental element is removed altogether."

The second of these two fundamental objections is that, in order to secure a conviction for the offence of indirect discrimination, the prosecution is not required to prove the guilt of defendants "beyond reasonable doubt." Indeed, it is now sufficient first to establish that the members of some racially defined set[7] are either less than proportionately represented in some enviable sort of occupation, association, or achievement, or disproportionately over-represented in some unenviable occupation, association, or form of achievement. This done, it is the defendants who now, if they are to escape conviction, have to prove their innocence; again, presumably, "beyond reasonable doubt."

This presumption of racially discriminatory guilt is obnoxious on two counts. In the first place, and generally, it is obnoxious for the same reason as any other presumption of criminal guilt must be. It is obnoxious, that is to say, in its abandonment of what has been one of the fundamental principles of British, and of course also of American, criminal law. As Richard Epstein, who describes himself as originally "a common law lawyer" (Ibid., p. xi) reasonably asks: "Why should the (assumed) importance of the anti-discrimination laws require us to slight the errors of over-enforcement? The consensus that murder is a grave wrong has never been regarded as a reason to make life easy for prosecutors: they do not get convictions on mere suspicion alone, or even on proof by a preponderance of the evidence. Quite the opposite" (Ibid., p. 225).

In the second place, the same presumption is obnoxious, more particularly, in the inadequacy of the evidence actually required for it to be received as established. For it to become highly probable that defendants actually are guilty of hostile racist discrimination against members of a certain racial set, it has got to be the case that, absent such discrimination, it would be reasonable to expect members of that particular set to be more or less proportionately represented among those selected for appointments, promotions, awards, or whatever else is the subject of litigation.

We should, however, in order to justify that expectation need to make an enormous assumption for which, it seems, evidence is rarely requested and never supplied. That assumption is that, as between the different racially and/or culturally defined sets in question, and in respect of whatever are the inherited and/or acquired characteristics that contribute to objective suitability for the forms of employment in question, there are *even on average* no significant differences across those entire sets.

That emphatic qualification "on average" is crucially important, for two very different reasons. In the first place, to say that something happens a certain way *on average* is not to say that it happens that way *every time*. But discussion about affirmative action and litigation about disparate impact usually proceeds on the assumption that there is no such thing as statistical variance. If Hispanics are 8 percent of the carpenters in a given town it does not follow that *every* employer of carpenters in that town would, if there were no discrimination either friendly or hostile, employ 8 percent Hispanics. Even if carpenters were assigned to employers by drawing lots there would be *variance* from one employer to another. Some employers would be employing more and some would be employing fewer than 8 percent Hispanics. To convict those employers with fewer Hispanics of hostile discrimination in hiring would be to make statistical variance a federal offence.

The second reason why the qualification "*on average*" is so vitally important is that it blocks certain inferences that might otherwise be legitimate. For if, and surely only if, it actually were the case that every member of some particular racial set was known to lack some characteristic essential to some kind of occupation or to some form of achievement, would membership of that particular racial set for that reason become a properly relevant, indeed a properly decisive, ground of disqualification. But if, as surely is in fact the case, there is no, or less than no, good experiential reason for believing that there is any racial set, all of the members of which both lack and lack the possibility of acquiring the characteristics essential to any particular kind of occupation or form of achievement, then no racial ground for disqualification for that particular kind of occupation or form of achievement can ever be legitimate.

The enormous and, as we have been urging, quite unwarranted assumption that, as between any different racially and/or culturally defined sets, there are no significant differences *even on average* in respect of either hereditarily given or acquirable and acquired employment- or achievement-relevant characteristics is not needed in order to justify Dr. Bunche's demand that the often very different claims of different individuals should be considered without regard to the racial set membership of those individuals.

The question of truth or falsity of that assumption becomes relevant only if and insofar as the very different ideal of racial equality it is sought to realize is: not that of a color-blind society in which all individuals are judged on their own individual merits and irrespective of their racial set membership; but instead that of an equality between racially defined collectives, the members of which see themselves and are to be seen not as individuals achieving or failing to achieve on their own individual merits or demerits, but rather as individuals representing the racial "communities" of which they see themselves, and wish to be seen, as members. It was, as will soon become very clear, an ill-omened day for all of us who, like Dr. Bunche, want to live in racially mixed yet *truly* color-blind societies when, in 1965, the U.S. Department of Labor, without any reference to supporting evidence but on its own sheer authority, pronounced that:

> Intelligence potential is distributed among Negro infants in the same proportion and pattern as among Icelanders or Chinese, or any other group. There is absolutely no question of any genetic differential.

Anti-Discriminatory Welfare Rights Actually Promote Discrimination

Because Epstein was, in his 1992 *Forbidden Grounds*, concerned with employment discrimination in general, rather than with racist discrimination in particular, his emphasis throughout was upon how such laws and regulations restrict civil rights to freedom of contract, and in consequence burden the economy. It is both instructive and important to bring out also that and how measures originally intended to outlaw racist discrimination tend, it would seem inexorably and in the not very long run, to extend and institutionalize, albeit in a new form, the very evil they were introduced to outlaw.

It would seem that the word "racist," like the word "fascist," has come to be used, especially by those most eager to employ it, as a vehemently emotive term of abuse, but often one with precious little if any determinate descriptive meaning. Yet, it only becomes properly a term of abuse insofar as it is construed to refer to a sort of behavior; namely, the advantaging or disadvantaging of individuals for no other and better reason than that they belong to this particular racial set and not that. Such behavior is (almost) always wrong since it is (almost) always unjustly irrelevant to the employment and other discriminations that are at issue.[8]

To all of us for whom the repudiation of racism, in this understanding, is a matter of principle, rather than a question of whose ox it is that is being gored, it is immediately obvious that the criminalization of "disparate impact" and of "indirect discrimination" tends very strongly to promote paradigm cases of racism in the form of "positive discrimination," "race norming," and "racial quotas." For how else but by engaging in these manifestly racist practices are employers and other appointers and awarders to secure themselves against conviction for committing these new pretendedly but not genuinely racist offences?

The whole experience, first of the U.S. and then of the UK, makes it absolutely clear that the way to reduce racist discrimination to insignificance is not the way of criminalization and quangos (quasi-autonomous non-government organizations) such as the EEOC and its British equivalent the Commission for Racial Equality (CRE).[9] On the contrary: that is the Royal Road not to a color-blind but to a "racially sensitive" and hence to a racially obsessed society.

The nearest the UK ever came to having the sort of debate that, as Richard Epstein rightly regrets, never occurred in the USA was in the Parliamentary debates on the Bill that became the Race Relations Act 1976. That was not very near. So it is important to stress here something that certainly would have been stressed had such a general debate ever occurred in the UK. It is that the UK, unlike, of course, the USA, had no history either of slavery or of its abolition followed by extensive institutionalized discrimination against blacks. On the contrary, a popular movement among the British people played the leading part in achieving first the abolition of the slave trade and later the emancipation of all the slaves in the then very extensive British dominions overseas. That these were genuinely popular movements can be shown by quoting from two letters. The first quotation is taken from a letter dated August 1814, written by the then British Foreign Secretary to the British Ambassador in Madrid:

> ...You must really press the Spanish Government to give us some more facilities on the subject of [the Abolition of] the Slave Trade, else we can do nothing for them, however well inclined: the nation is bent upon this object. I believe there is hardly a village that has not met and petitioned upon it; both Houses of Parliament are pledged to press it; and the Ministers must make it the basis of their policy.[10]

The second quotation is taken from a letter written in 1862 by the then U.S. Ambassador in London:

> The Emancipation Proclamation has done more for us here than all our former victories and all our diplomacy. It is creating an almost convulsive reaction in our favour all over this country...public opinion is very deeply stirred here and finds expression in meetings, addresses to President Lincoln, deputations to us, standing committees to agitate the subject and to affect opinion, and all the other symptoms of a great popular movement.[11]

The status of slavery had of course never been recognized by the English Common Law. I will not refrain from quoting some concluding words from the 1777 Judgement of Lord Mansfield, Chief Justice of England, in the case of an imported slave:

> The air of England has long been too pure for a slave, and every man who breathes it. Every man who comes into England is entitled to the protection of English law, whatever oppression he may heretofore have suffered, and whatever may be the colour of his skin.

Despite and/or because of this very different historical background there certainly was in the UK both more stubborn color-prejudice and more principled rejection of such prejudice than in most other

European countries, simply because a much larger proportion of the British people had either visited or lived for a substantial part of their working lives in parts of those pre-World War II extensive overseas British dominions that were—and of course still are—populated by non-white peoples.[12]

The British Race Relations Act 1976 was introduced after about twenty-five years of fairly substantial immigration first of blacks, mainly from the West Indies; and then, a little later, of what quickly became and always remained a much larger number of browns, mainly from the Indian sub-continent. It was introduced because there was no question but that a lot of hostile discrimination was occurring (by no means all of it by whites against non-whites) and because, although the proportion of non-whites in the total population was at that time extremely small, and even now is not more than 7 percent, that minority was, or those minorities were, from the beginning concentrated in relatively few areas.

I suspect, but without first unearthing and then reading the relevant pages of Hansard I cannot hope to prove, that the main reason why the Race Relations Bill contained clauses mandating the establishment of the CRE was a widespread recognition that there would be a deal of difficulty in discovering, much less proving, any but the most obvious and flagrant cases of hostile discrimination. Its passage into law did indeed cause these cases to disappear almost as quickly as the passage into law of the U.S. Civil Rights Act 1964 had caused their American equivalents to disappear.

There was, however, a possible reason for not stopping legislative action in the UK once this was achieved, but proceeding to establish the CRE; one possible reason that did not apply in the USA. It was that there were then in the UK many—as there still are, but substantially fewer—nationalized industries, which, being translated, are, or were, state monopoly producers and providers of goods and services. Such monopolists were, necessarily, free from the pressures of competition. So whereas firms operating in ordinary competitive markets without legal protection against the entry of rivals will, if they persist in preferring to hire workers for reasons irrelevant to the performance of the work in question, necessarily incur costs their less prejudiced competitors avoid, monopolistic firms will not. Firms operating in competitive markets therefore have a strong self-interest in eschewing occupationally irrelevant grounds of discrimination not only in their hiring and firing but also in their buying and selling and in all other business dealings.[13]

At the time of writing, the UK and all the other subordinate member states of the European Union (EU) were in process of obediently adopting a Charter of Fundamental Rights. While this Charter enumerates most of the fundamental civil, political, and economic liberties that are at the foundation of any free society, these are all threatened by the incorporation into this Charter of an additional array of redistributive welfare rights that must necessarily increase the already inordinate tax and regulatory burdens on producers, and reduce the resources available for productive investment in the EU.[14] In the UK, the Blair administration from its beginning significantly insisted on obscuring the importance of productive investment by systematically misdescribing as investment all state spending on state-provided welfare services.

Nor should anyone familiar with the actual operation and achievements of either the EEOC or the CRE be surprised to learn that, under the Burden of Proof Directive of the EU, anyone who is accused of any form of legally recognized employment discrimination is to be presumed *guilty* until and unless they succeed in proving—to the satisfaction of the court—their innocence. Very understandably, but not for that reason excusably, it seems never to occur to the EEOC or the CRE, or to any of their opposite numbers that may have been established in other countries, that the difficulty of proving the offence might arise from the fact that it had not in truth actually been committed.

Race, Culture, and Intelligence

Perhaps the most profitable way of elucidating the relations and lacks of relations between the concepts of race, culture, and intelligence is by considering the mistreatment of these matters in Ken Richardson and David Spears' (Eds.) *Race, Culture and Intelligence* (London, Penguin,[15] 1972). That was a work that seems to have had an enormous and wholly unfortunate influence, especially upon both those studying and those teaching in departments, colleges, schools, and institutes of education.[16]

In their "Editorial Foreword," the Editors of this book claim that they "have attempted to step back from the debate itself and look at the concepts which underlie it." But the book is in the event so far from containing "the close examination of the key ideas" that is also promised in that "Editorial Foreword" that no contributor, from beginning to end, can spare a moment from execrating reactionaries and racists in order to spell out either what it is to be a racist or why racism is wrong.

After this no one will be surprised, though they may well still be shocked, to learn that none of the contributors to a work professedly dealing with the controversial topics of *Race, Culture and Intelligence* thought it necessary to provide a definition of the word "culture." So no one brings out the crucial difference between, on the one hand, race, which most certainly is genetically determined, and, on the other hand, culture which, equally certainly, is not. The contributor who comes nearest to doing this—and it is not exactly close—is Donald Swift, Professor of Education at the Open University. His contribution is entitled "What is the Environment?" In it he announces: "And finally we cannot accept quality distinctions between cultures" (p. 156).

He appears not to have noticed that this remarkable confession of incapacity must disqualify him from maintaining, what, as a Professor of Education he is surely required at least to pretend to believe, that it is better to be well educated than ill educated or not educated at all. Even more embarrassing for him should be his consequent disqualification from sincerely and with understanding asserting that any culture that is racist or sexist is, at least in those respects, worse than one that is neither.

The first necessities here are to distinguish between high and low cultures and between intrinsic and instrumental good. In the broad sense beloved of professing social scientists, the culture of a social set comprises not only its high culture, if any—its music, literature, arts, science, and so on—but also its language, its mating and child-raising practices, its religious and other traditions, its official and its actual values, and on down through the whole long list of the professional interests of anthropologists and sociologists. An intrinsic value is something that is believed to be good in itself. Something is said to have instrumental value in so far as it is good for producing something else.

That some cultures can be and are for some purposes instrumentally better than others is a proposition that was categorically and definitively proved to be true by the findings of the research work reported in Thomas Sowell *Ethnic America* (New York: Basic Books, 1981). In this research Sowell followed the track records of nine different sets of immigrants from the time of their first arrival until they became assimilated. The differences between the cultures from and with which they came go a very long way in explaining the sometimes quite spectacular differences in the nature and extent of their subsequent achievements.

Perhaps the most memorable example of all such differences is provided in a rather later work, Sowell 1984: "Back before World War I, a study in New York City showed that German and Jewish school children graduated from high school at a rate more than a hundred times that for Irish and Italian children" (p. 38). Now that really was, for the Irish and Italian children, an achievement in under-achievement! Nor, in view of the later rises of both Irish-Americans and Italian-Americans, is it plausible to try to diminish this negative achievement by postulating any genetically determined inferiorities.

In *Race, Culture and Intelligence*, a work in which, as we have seen, the editors at one point claim that "they have attempted to step back from the debate itself and look at the concepts which underlie it," the "Editorial Foreword" begins with a two sentence paragraph. Having now come to realize that neither the editors nor any of their other contributors actually even attempted to define any of the key terms in the debate, we should not be surprised to find that that paragraph provides a partisan misrepresentation of "the debate itself." It reads:

> This collection of essays about intelligence stems from the revived nature-nurture controversy about the origins of mental abilities, led notably by Arthur Jensen, and more recently by H. J. Eysenck in Britain. Their position, ostensibly vindicated by dispassionate appeal to scientific evidence, attributes the persistent IQ differences between U.S. blacks and whites predominantly to differences in genetic constitution.

What this paragraph suggests is that what first Jensen and later Eysenck were maintaining was that all blacks are inferior to all whites in IQ. What they actually were maintaining was a totally different thing, with totally different implications. It was that there is *on average* a substantial difference in IQ between the class of all blacks and the class of all whites, hence the title of *The Bell Curve* for that much abused work Herrnstein and Murray 1994.

The only contributors to *Race, Culture and Intelligence* who provide readers with a usable reference to the paper that expounds what

Professor Donald Swift sees as "the blinkered scientism of the Jensenist heresy" (p. 156) are Martin Richards, Ken Richardson, and David Spears. They do it in, curiously, a final article, "Conclusions: Intelligence and Society." They there list, as "Further Reading," A. R. Jensen "How much can we boost IQ and scholastic achievement?" *Harvard Educational Review*, vol. 39, No. 1, 1969 (p. 145).

The publication of this Jensen article occasioned a coast-to-coast brouhaha.[17] That monstrously misnamed and hopefully long since defunct outfit Students for a Democratic Society (SDS) sponsored a wave of tire-slashing, slogan-painting, telephoned or shouted abuse and threats, and strident demands to "Fire" or even to "Kill Jensen." The campaign went on to embrace two further favourite enemies: the Harvard psychologist Richard Herrnstein, co-author of *IQ in the Meritocracy*, and, a little out of place, the Nobel Prize-winning physicist, William Shockley.

The spillover into the UK included a happily not very severe physical assault on the psychologist H. J. Eysenck at the London School of Economics. This was one of several exercises in the implementation of a policy introduced by the National Union of Students (NUS) in the academic year 1969-70. That policy was "by all available means" to prevent any meeting in any British institution of tertiary education being addressed by a speaker deemed by the local NUS branch to be "racist or fascist." In all the years in which the NUS maintained this outrageously illiberal policy it was, so far as I know, never possible—and some of us tried very persistently—to extract from any NUS spokesperson a definition of the word "racism" under which it was clearly true both that racist behavior is morally wrong and that the intended victim of the no-platform policy was an advocate of racist behavior.

That no-platform policy, adopted over thirty years ago, has long since been abandoned. But the "closed" (i.e., secret) member of the Communist Party who was president of the National Union of Students for the academic years 1969-70 and 1970-71 became Home Secretary for the whole period of the first Blair administration (1997-2001). In that period he was responsible first for appointing Sir William Macpherson of Cluny to conduct an inquiry into the circumstances and the investigation of the supposedly racist murder of a young black named Stephen Lawrence, and then later responsible for wholeheartedly and unreservedly accepting the resulting Report.

That Report, almost universally known simply as *The Macpherson Report*,[18] is also almost universally taken to have demonstrated that all the major UK institutions are infected with institutional racism, and hence that they urgently require institutional disinfection. Macpherson himself obviously believed that his Report succeeded in demonstrating these desired conclusions. Yet one searches it in vain for evidence that any of the actions or statements of any officer in the Metropolitan Police Service (MPS) was racist, in the sense of the word "racist" defined on page 81, above. Indeed, whenever concrete evidential matters are at stake there are clear exonerations of the individual officers in question.[19] Again, the *Report* expresses anxiety lest it should be misunderstood. Was it saying that the policies of the MPS were racist? No. "It is vital for us to stress that neither academic debate nor the evidence presented to us leads us to say or conclude that an accusation that institutional racism exists in the MPS implies that the policies of the MPS are racist. No such evidence is before us. Indeed the contrary is true."[20]

The *Report* nevertheless reaches from its study—only of the MPS—the astoundingly comprehensive conclusion that not only the MPS but also all the other major institutions of the United Kingdom are similarly infected with institutional racism. So far as I can see we are not anywhere in all the 325 pages of this enormous *Report* provided with any explicit explanation of how this central and crucial conclusion was reached. But it surely must have been by the application everywhere of its own peculiar definition of "a racist incident," a definition that it insists "should be universally adopted by the Police, local Government and other relevant agencies."[21]

That recommended definition reads: "A racist incident is *any* incident which is perceived to be racist by the victim or *any* other person."[22] So, it appears that, in the nightmare world of criminal justice according to Sir William Macpherson of Cluny, any incident, not just any crime, involving any person from any minority of "color, ethnic origin, or culture," is a racist incident if anyone at all, whether from that minority or from the majority, chooses to say that it is. And if this outrageously preposterous and potentially explosive recommendation was not by itself more than sufficiently damaging, it is immediately followed by the equally imperative recommendation—directed at the police!—that the expression "racist incident" is one that "must be understood to include crimes and *non crimes* in policing terms. Both must be reported, recorded and investigated with equal commitment."[23]

Perhaps the most remarkable and certainly the most sinister feature of the entire Macpherson inquiry was the fact that, despite their admitted innocence of any individual racist guilt, all the police officers called to testify were required to "recognise and accept" the "fact," and themselves publicly to declare, that their own conduct was the cause of dissatisfaction with and justified hostility to the police. Failure to publicly declare their guilt could result only from "their lack of understanding" of "the essential problem and its depth." This "essential problem" clearly was, although that is not actually stated at this point, institutional racism.[24]

Such inquisitorial proceedings ought to remind anyone with any knowledge of twentieth-century history of the abject false confessions required and made in the Stalinist show trials, first in Moscow in 1936, and subsequently in the various countries added to the Soviet Empire after World War II.[25]

The *Macpherson Report* provides no definition of the expression "institutional racism"[26] and gives no reason why those employed in an institution correctly characterized as being institutionally racist should feel guilty about their professional involvement in that institution. What apparently leads to the conclusion "that not only the MPS but also all other major institutions in the United Kingdom are…infected with institutional racism" is—although it is never actually said in these very words—that these institutions have what the EEOC in the USA would call a disparate impact on racial minorities. This technical expression, being interpreted, means that members of racial minority sets are proportionately under-represented in whatever is enviable about the affairs of these institutions and/or over-represented in whatever about those affairs is unenviable. In the case of the MPS the enviable are presumably its employees and the unenviable convicted criminals.

We have been concerned here primarily, if not only, with the unsoundness of arguments from such proportionate over- and under-representations to racist discrimination as its cause. In the case of the MPS the proportionate under-representation of blacks is certainly substantial and might well be largely if not wholly explained as due to hostile racist discrimination. But the proportionate over-representation of blacks among the convicted criminals is so enormous as to make Jack Straw's attempt to dismiss it with references to "institutional racism" a dereliction from his duty as minister of state at the Home Office.

The 1999 *Statistics on Race and the Criminal Justice System*, issued by the Home Office only after the publication of *The Macpherson Report*, provides some astonishing figures. But first you have to wade through the statutory Foreword by Jack Straw telling us that we must learn the lessons of *The Macpherson Report*, and purge the criminal justice system of "institutional racism." Then we have another Foreword by Mr. Justice Rose, chairman of the Criminal Justice Consultative Committee, stating that we must learn the lessons of *The Macpherson Report* and purge the criminal justice system of "institutional racism." Then—surprise, surprise!—we have an insert from the Commission for Racial Equality telling us we must learn the lessons of *The Macpherson Report* and purge the criminal justice system of "institutional racism."

It is only half way down Table 7.5 on page 44 that we get any hard data. If we remember that only 2 percent of the UK population is black we ought to be astonished to read that, as of June 30, 1998, 7.1 percent of those serving prison sentences for burglary were black. For the same date the figure for theft and handling was 7.5 percent, for sexual offences 8.1 percent, for violence against the person 9.7 percent, for fraud and forgery 13.2 percent, for drug offences 19 percent, and for robbery 22.6 percent.

Two final things need to be said here before concluding this section. One is that the degree of the over-representation of young blacks among those who have committed crimes is comparable with the degree of their over-representation among those who, as the sons of single mothers, have presumably suffered the effects of a fatherless upbringing. On this, compare chapter 3, above. The other is to wonder whether the Jack Straw who so uncritically and so enthusiastically accepted the recommendations of *The Macpherson Report* has learned anything at all about the actual nature of racism and the practical difficulties and implications of attempts to combat it by political measures since, all those long years ago, he was president of the NUS.

Welfare Rights for the Brutes?

It was in 1776, a year during which the United Kingdom's American colonists had very different interests in the fronts of their minds, that Dr. Johnson remarked that he was hearing "much talk of the misery which we cause the brute creation." Certainly there were at about that time several relevant publications. Today it perhaps needs to be explained that in Catholic Christianity, both Roman and Anglo, the brutes are all non-human animals: that is to say, those kinds of animals of which the material bodies are not supposed to be occupied and managed by separable immaterial and immortal souls. The first Act of Parliament directed to reducing the miseries of any of these brutes was passed in 1822. The Royal Society for the Prevention of Cruelty to Animals (RSPCA) was founded two years later, in 1824. A further growth of such concern, focusing initially on anti-vivisection, began in the early 1870s and lasted roughly forty years. Its first legislative achievement was the passage of the Cruelty to Animals Act in 1876. Its last was the passage of the Protection of Animals Act in 1911.

During and between the wars the work of the RSPCA of course continued. But it seems that legislative changes were neither achieved nor very strenuously attempted. During the first twenty-five years after World War II there were four official enquiries—into blood sports, live exports, modern farming, and animal experimentation—and the National Anti-Vivisection Society (NAVS) and the League Against Cruel Sports (LACS) persuaded backbench Members of Parliament (MPs) to introduce various always-aborted Private Members' Bills. But from then on, what had traditionally been called the animal welfare movement began to grow, and to change very substantially. From being middle class, non-political, and predominantly female and elderly, it became classless, youthful, and politically activist. It grew to be a substantial element in what Peter Simple used to call the protest industry. As a movement it now concentrates on the institutionalized evils of factory farming, animal experimentation, and wildlife exploitation rather than the mistreatment of domestic pets.

For us, what is most relevant in this development was the introduction of claims that brutes have rights. The development of these claims is to be attributed to a group of philosophers working in Oxford in the 1970s—Andrew Linzey, Stephen Clark and, a little later, Peter Singer. But the original identification and labeling of the new sin of speciesism was the achievement of a social scientist, Richard Ryder.[27]

Any philosophical inquiry into rights has to begin by making three crucial distinctions, two of which have been noticed already. The first is between moral rights and legal rights. Since legal rights are created by and maintained under some particular system of law, it is possible for some individual or set of individuals to have, under that system, either a legal right to something to which they have no moral right, or a moral right to something to which they have no legal right. The second distinction is between option and welfare rights. Option rights are rights to be left free to choose. Welfare rights are rights to be supplied with some good, presumably either by some other person or persons or by some organization. The third distinction is between artificial and natural rights. Legal rights are all, as such and necessarily, artificial, since they are created and maintained under some particular system of law. But it is also possible for individuals to artificially create moral rights. For instance, by promising to give someone some specific sum of money if they fulfill certain specified conditions I thereby endow them with a moral right to receive that sum of money from me if they satisfy those conditions. The classic proclamation of natural rights that are at the same time option rights was, as we have seen, made in the American Declaration of Independence.

No doubt all those who maintain that all or some of the brutes possess rights also want those rights to become rights recognized and maintained by the state. But it is by insisting upon their being, in the first instance, moral that they hope to achieve that objective. So, since these moral rights are supposedly possessed by all the members either of the set of all brutes or of some of its subsets, the protagonists of animal rights are in effect issuing a declaration of the universal moral rights of all the members of another, non-human, kind of individuals.

But how is this declaration itself to be justified? If we were to construe the Declaration of Independence, as no doubt many of the Signers themselves did, as asserting that the Creator had endowed all men with certain unalienable rights by a direct act of the Divine will, then this assertion would be open to the objection that rights prescribed by the positive law of the Creator or of any other being or institution would, necessarily and as such, be legal rather than moral. The heart of this particular matter of logic was first laid bare in Plato's *Euthyphro*: if you define the moral in terms of the will of God you thereby disclaim all possibility of rendering substantial and non-tautological praise to God for the Divine Goodness.[28]

So what is to be done? The first step must be to insist that the moral rights proclaimed in that great Declaration, moral rights the validity of which the supporters of liberalizing legal reforms in the UK often appealed to during the 1960s, should not be construed, as critics nowadays often pretend that they were then construed, as being moral rights for everyone to do whatever they might choose to do regardless of the harm they would inflect on others by so doing.

Since, according to that great Declaration, everyone is endowed with equal rights, the rights of every individual must in consequence be limited by the subsistence of the corresponding and equivalent rights of everyone else. It is this essential restriction that provides a basis for the contention that in asserting these equal rights of all men or, better, all human persons—could there be non-human or non-physical persons?—we are at one and the same time asserting both our own rights and our corresponding duties to others.

The subsistence of these logically necessary connections should have become manifest from our consideration of the rationale behind the Declaration. For just as no individual human being in a State of Nature could have any right to prescribe an item for inclusion in a system of Laws of Nature unless he simultaneously accepted a reciprocal obligation himself to obey that prescription, so no individuals can reasonably claim a right to a liberty or indeed to anything else unless they are prepared simultaneously to accept an obligation to respect the corresponding rights of everyone else.

It is, surely, a presupposition of the rationale provided for the origin of the natural moral rights proclaimed in the Declaration of Independence that no set of living creatures can properly be described as having moral rights unless it is a set whose members are not only able to claim those rights for themselves simply as members of that set, but also to recognize corresponding and consequential duties to the other members of that same set. Can anyone suggest any other way of justifying the contention that the universal option rights proclaimed in the American Declaration of Independence are indeed moral rights? For better or for worse, this justification—and what other is available?—rules out all possibility of moral rights for any of the brutes.

This rationale for the possession of moral option rights has the great merit of exposing the outrageousness of claims to possess supposedly moral welfare rights—rights that apparently impose no corresponding duties upon their possessors. Insistence upon the outrageousness of such claims has, as was argued earlier, its greatest relevance in the context of discussion about radical reform of welfare states.

All this might perhaps seem to be, if not formally and strictly, at least in some way inconsistent with an eagerness to insist that we do have duties to at least some of the brutes. But it is not. For to insist that we can and do have some duties to some of the brutes is perfectly consistent with maintaining that, because they do not and cannot have duties either to other members of their own species or to members of ours, they do not and cannot have rights to our executing any of our duties to them.

Perhaps the popular line of argument for the conclusion that at least some of the brutes have rights begins by pointing out that the members of the set of this favored some are endowed with characteristics in embryonic form that are, in more developed forms, considered to be peculiarly and distinctively human. From this observation the argument proceeds, by way of the suggestion that the difference between human beings and the brutes is a mere difference of degree, to the desired conclusion that it is simply not possible to draw a sharp, clear line between one category and the other.

That it should be possible to find most of what have been taken to be defining characteristics of humanity among the brutes—at least in some embryonic form—is of course implied by general evolutionary theory. But before dismissing all differences of degree as *mere* differences of degree we should consider what is meant by a "difference of degree" and look at one or two other examples of such differences.

Let us say that difference of degree between two extremes is one in which there is a series of actual or theoretically possible cases stretching between one of these extremes and the other, and with the amount of difference between each member of the series and the next vanishingly small. It now becomes obvious that differences that are large, as well as differences of degree, can be of the most enormous human importance. For the differences, for instance, between age and youth, sanity and insanity, a free society and one in which everything that is not forbidden is compulsory, are all of enormous human importance, yet at the same time are differences of degree in the sense explained.

In the present case it really is, although the differences between the embryonic and developed forms of the defining characteristics of humanity are all differences of degree, unusually easy to draw a sharp, clear line between the distinctively human and the distinctively non-human.

There are two reasons for this. The first is that there are several characteristics that have been suggested as defining, and all of these need to be present if a being is to be accepted as unequivocally human. The second reason is that some of the relevant differences of degree are very large indeed. Thus, for instance, there is huge difference between the most sophisticated communication systems employed by any non-human species and the most primitive of human natural languages. Certainly no such non-human communication system is equipped with the concepts that would make it possible for those who employ it to use it either to claim rights as members of their own species or to recognize their corresponding and consequential duties to their fellow members.

I have so far been arguing, perhaps somewhat impatiently, both that all of us human beings are by our rational natures endowed with moral rights and that the brutes are as such disqualified from enjoying a similar endowment. I nevertheless wholeheartedly agree with Jeremy Bentham—who had no time for any notion of rights—about what it is that makes them proper objects of moral concern: "The question is not can they reason or can they talk, but can they suffer?"

Indeed they can. And certainly it is a possibility that has been, and despite all the efforts of animal welfare movements, continues to be, far too abundantly realized. The prime motive of all animal welfare movements has always been, and surely still remains, compassion rather than a concern to secure and promote the putative rights of non-human animals.

Notes

1. In my copy the text fills six printed pages.
2. It was because of "his peculiar felicity of expression" that the Continental Congress chose young Mr. Jefferson to produce the final draft.
3. Calls for "preferential hiring" as the means to achieve proportionate representation can be found in, for instance, *Testament of Hope: The Essential Writings of Martin Luther King, Jr.* (San Francisco: Harper and Row, 1986). Compare Rockwell, Llewelyn H., "The Economics of Martin Luther King Jr.," in *The Free Market*, February 1991.
4. The first British formulation of this sociological law was provoked by the activities of the Commission for Racial Equality (CRE), established under the UK Race Relations Act 1976. For more about the particular problems which that organization has done so much to exaggerate and so little solve, see, for instance, Honeyford, Ray, 1999. It should not here go unremarked that it was only after offering this book to ten or more UK publishers, and meeting in every case a firm rejection, that the author sought and found acceptance in the USA.
5. Compare, for instance, D'Souza 1991 and Kors and Silvergate 1998.
6. In the UK this is the highest legal office, which is always filled by a leading professional lawyer. On appointment such lawyers automatically become, if not already, peers of the realm.
7. By Cantor's Axiom for Sets the sole essential feature of a set is that its members have at least one common characteristic, any kind of characteristic. The comparative advantage of the word "set" is that, unlike such words as "class," it lacks all particular implications.
8. The parenthetical qualifications are needed in order to admit, for instance, the choice of a black actor to play the part of Othello and a white actress that of Desdemona.
9. It, together with the subordinate institutions that proliferated since its establishment, has been, with Hastie's Law in mind, nicknamed "The Race Relations Industry." See Wharton, Michael, 1999.
10. Borrowed from Russell, Bertrand, *Freedom and Organisation: 1914-1904* (London: Allen and Unwin, 1934), p. 41.
11. Borrowed from Carl Sandburg's biography of Abraham Lincoln, Vol. II, chapter 13.
12. My own wife was born and lived in Burma until at the age of eleven she had to fly out before the advancing Japanese Army. Her father later walked out through the roadless jungle into Assam, afterwards returning with the victorious British XIVth Army.
13. That is why the editors of the notorious Nazi (National Socialist German Workers' Party) antisemitic and anti-capitalist weekly *Der Stürmer* used in almost every issue to publish cartoons attacking the racial insensitivity of business persons for whom payments from any source were equally welcome.
14. The importance of these tax and regulatory burdens on producers is revealed by the comparative positions of the main EU countries on the Index of Economic Freedoms. Germany stands at No. 20, Italy at No. 29, and France at No. 45. Before the Blair administration adopted the Social Charter and the Working Time Directive, the UK was, along with the U.S. and five other English-speaking countries, among the top ten. But even before the latest increases in UK taxation it had fallen to No. 11 and, as its tax rates are progressively "harmonized" upwards to EU levels, it will fall much further.
15. In fairness to a firm that has over the years provided an enormously valuable service to the English-speaking public round the world by making cheap paperback reprints

of so many worthy books, it should perhaps be noted that the imprint on the title page is not that of Penguin Books but of Penguin Education. That particular and long since dissolved subsection of the Penguin Books organization had, and fully deserved, a reputation as a producer of hard left propaganda. See, for one index of its inspirational achievements, note 17, below.

16. It is an occasion to quote Thomas Sowell's observation: "Education is a notoriously undemanding field of study" (Sowell 1986, p. 160). That was an observation that often came to my mind while working on Flew 1987, a book that dealt with the decline of the maintained school system in the UK and the reasons for that decline.

17. There is an account of its spill-over into the UK in Flew 1976, chapter 5. The main victims of such assaults were H. J. Eysenck and the sometime headmaster Ray Honeyford. The best account of the whole business on both sides of the Atlantic is Pearson, Roger, *Race, Intelligence and Bias in Academe* (Washington: Scott-Townsend, 1991). In it we find a quotation from Eysenck, which in the present context provides a salutary read:

    What upset me more than anything...was the fact that my children were made to suffer by their teachers, whose Left-Wing views led them to vent their outrage at my (alleged) views on the innocent. Whenever my name got into the papers, they would make pointed remarks in class, putting my children in an impossible position. *Things got so bad that I changed my name by deed poll to Evans; this afforded the children some protection, particularly later when they went on to University* (pp. 38-9; emphasis added.)

18. *The Stephen Lawrence Inquiry: Report of an Inquiry by Sir William Macpherson of Cluny* (London: Stationery office, 2000). Anyone inclined to accept the conclusions of this Report ought to study Green, David G. (ed.), 2000; also Dennis, Norman, Erdos, George, and Al-slahi, Ahmed 2000.

19. *Macpherson Report*, pp. 51-2, 52-3, and 54.

20. Ibid., p. 24.

21. Ibid., p. 329.

22. Ibid., p. 328 (emphases added).

23. Ibid., p. 329 (emphasis added).

24. Ibid., p. 8.

25. See, for a development of this analogy, Ellis, Frank, 2001.

26. Sir William Macpherson of Cluny would surely be both astonished and embarrassed were he ever to learn what the purposes of the "black power" militant Stokely Carmichael (later Kwame Ture) were in introducing this concept. See Horowitz, David, 1999, pp. 81, 204, and 214-5.

27. He produced his leaflet *Speciesism* in Oxford in 1970.

28. See, for a development of this argument Flew, Antony, 1971, pp. 26-33.

6

Sincerity, Rationality, and Monitoring

It is a mark of insincerity of purpose to seek the Sacred Emperor in low-class teashops.
—Words uttered by Kai Lung the storyteller, in Ernest Bramah, The Wallet of Kai Lung

In the case imagined by Kai Lung, the insincerity of purpose would have been at once obvious to everyone. But, in order to detect and display the insincerity of purpose that is so often to be found both in the operations of tax-funded organizations and in the operations of those who are employed by such organizations, it is necessary first to achieve a vivid appreciation of the logically necessary linkages between the related concepts of sincerity of purpose, rationality in the pursuit of purposes, and the monitoring of success or failure in the achievement of purposes pursued.

Three Basic Principles

The first and most manifest principle that has here to be firmly grasped is that anyone sincerely and rationally pursuing any objectives whatsoever—objectives good or bad, large or small, particular or general—must be constantly concerned to monitor their success or failure in approaching and attaining those objectives.

Suppose first—to begin in a remarkable if somewhat eccentric way—that someone proclaims to have embarked upon a Quest for the Holy Grail. And suppose that, almost as soon as the fanfares have died, that person settles for the first antique-seeming mug offered by the first fluent rogue in the local bazaar. Then we surely have to say that this neglect of any serious and systematic enquiry, this total lack of interest either in the history of the purchase to be put in the place of honor on the mantelpiece, or in the evidence that the real thing does after all survive somewhere else, all conspire to show that, whatever else that particular someone was after, he most certainly could not have been sincerely trying to unearth and to acquire the vessel actually used in the original Last Supper. Sincerity of purpose thus absolutely presupposes a strong concern as to whether and how far the purpose entertained has been or is being achieved.

Again, suppose that some businesswoman has dared to declare her self-interested, and therefore in some eyes necessarily selfish, resolve to make an overall profit. But then suppose that she takes no steps to ensure that accounts are kept, revealing which parts of her operation are and are not making a profit. Then as before, we have no option but to conclude that, whatever her true aim may be, it is not making a profit. Perhaps she really is—as the stock phrase has it—in business for the sake of her health. Certainly, if she had been sincerely devoted to the pursuit of profit, she could not but have insisted upon the keeping of at least one set of books. (Had totally uninhibited profit maximization been the name of the game she might well have had a second set also—for the exclusive benefit of the Internal Revenue Service!)

The second principle is a corollary of the first. For a large part of the point of monitoring progress, or the lack of it, is in order to determine whether and when some alteration of approach is called for. So, especially in so far as those who assert that they are sincerely seeking to attain some particular objective have any claim to being even half-way rational, they have to be ready to change course by adopting fresh methods if ever and whenever their previous methods are in fact proving not to be producing that particular objective. Such adaptability, and such actual adaptation, surely is a large part of what we have in mind when we speak of intelligence and of rationality.

Let us, therefore, now apply this second principle to the first of the two illustrations. Its validity at once becomes apparent. Suppose that our proclaimed Seeker after the Holy Grail was confronted with, and accepted, a demonstration that the mug on the mantelpiece was not the genuine article. And suppose that, instead of renewing his quest, but in some different area, he was content with what he had. Then, presumably, we should have to conclude that he never had been sincere in his seeking, or at any rate that, even if he did start as a serious and sincere seeker, he is one no longer.

Suppose next, what is rather more interesting, that our pretended Grail Seeker, instead of attending to the discrediting demonstration, and accepting it as such, refused to listen. Or suppose that, having listened with impatience, he then refused to accept it as a demonstration. There are, of course, all manner of marginal and confusing possible cases here. But let us, in order to get the fundamentals straight, suppose an overwhelming and unequivocally valid demonstration.

Then, surely, people who show themselves to be altogether uninterested in and unaffected by that demonstration thereby reveal, in the most unambiguously clearcut way, either their total indifference as to whether the proposition thus demonstrated to be true is in fact true or it is in fact false, or their utter irrationality. We cannot but conclude either that our pretended Holy Grail Seeker was not sincerely seeking that object or that he was so totally irrational as to be incapable of the rational pursuit of any objective.

The third and last of the three principles is somewhat more complex than either of the first two, and maybe for that reason and others more controversial. It is this. In so far as any of the resources employed to secure the desired results are scarce—a condition that is always satisfied, even if the resources drawn on consist in nothing but the time and energy of those desiring those results—the purposers must, as rational beings, be concerned to achieve the maximum output of desired results in exchange for the minimum input of scarce resources. They must be so concerned. For, on the same assumptions of single-mindedness and sincerity of purpose, they cannot but want, by means of such greater economic efficiency, either to get more of those particular desired results from an unincreased investment of scarce resources, or else to obtain some or more of some other desired goods through an alternative investment of the surplus thereby saved.

We can, while continuing to operate at the same fairly high level of abstraction, draw out one further general yet very practical consequence from the conjunction of the first principle with this third. It is that those who are in truth both sincerely and single-mindedly devoted to the provision of some of all those enormously various goods that the ever-proliferating institutions of the welfare state are established and maintained to provide should have little difficulty in meeting the challenge the director of the Social Affairs Unit (SAU) put in the concluding paragraph of the chapter "Breaking the Spell of the Welfare State" in the SAU's first publication:

> Finally and most importantly, the welfare state distributes the burden of proof unfairly. All the earlier discussion about the requirements of an adequate criticism in an ideal debate rests upon a rather odd "given" assumption that it is up to the critic to prove that the welfare state is inadequate, or that one of its parts should be changed or cut, or that certain personnel should be sacked. This is clearly a ludicrous requirement to apply to some independent critic, an academic or a journalist. *It is the welfare state that consumes "public money"*[1] *and it is its obligation to prove that it is not wasting it.*[2]

It should be easy for all concerned to meet this challenge. For, as our first principle makes clear, precisely to the extent that they really are striving to achieve certain results perceived as good—results which no doubt are indeed truly good—they are bound already to be engaged in monitoring their own progress in achieving these ends. Given always the stated assumptions of good faith and minimal rationality, assumptions that those to whom these characteristics are attributed will scarcely wish to deny, it follows that they will know, and presumably be able to show to outside enquirers, what various goods it is they are succeeding in providing, and at least roughly how much of each they have managed to produce, and for what expenditure of resources.

It is not just useless—it is worse than useless—to respond by maintaining that some of the goods of human welfare are so intangible and so elusive that it is hard if not impossible to determine whether or where these goods have been attained. Hard it may be, and often is. But the problem of identification has got to be solved before anyone can begin to make any sincere and rational attempt to generate such admittedly intangible and elusive goods. To say that it is not just hard but downright impossible is to make a total nonsense of your whole enterprise. For to set yourself to strive to generate putative benefits of such a sort that it cannot be known whether anyone is enjoying these benefits or not is no more sensible than "The Hunting of the Snark"—an authentically fabulous creature which, it will be remembered, could not in principle have been identified even had it been found.[3]

The proper counter to any such pretentiously silly response is, surely, obvious.[4] Even if we allow, as perhaps in the present context we must, that it is unthinkable that any funds currently employed to finance any part of the welfare state apparatus should instead be left to individual citizens to spend as they individually see fit, still there will always be other parts of that apparatus that could and would use the resources bought by that funding to generate identifiable benefits—identifiable benefits, it should here perhaps be added, to be enjoyed by people other than those directly or indirectly employed by the welfare state apparatus itself.

A second, more sensible response is to complain that the goods actually generated, the benefits actually conferred, are far too miscellaneous to be summed into a single index of output. Certainly this is as true as it is important. How indeed could we even begin to construct such an unitary index of output—an index of output, that is, that was not a disguised reiteration of some less arbitrary index of resource input—for what has long since become Britain's, indeed Europe's,[5] largest employer, the National Health Service? But the truth and the importance of this observation in no way forecloses on the possibility, and the needs, not only to make economic efficiency calculations as between those different parts of the apparatus that are in fact directed at the same ends, but also to make hard decisions about the allocation of scarce resources as between the production of this health good or that.

Much as so many people would like to avoid such economic decisions and economic calculations, they cannot in fact be avoided. For, wherever and whenever scarce resources have possible alternative uses, economic decisions are inescapable. The truth is—and this is a logically necessary, definitional truth—that economic analysis deals with scarce means and various ends in general, rather than with any particular end or sort of ends to which those scarce resources are directed.[6]

Economic analyses, therefore, can find application wherever and whenever any kind of scarce resource is deployed to advance any sort of ends, however banausic or elevated those ends may be. They are not to be applied only to what are conventionally considered the wealth-creating elements in a national economy; or even to the economy only. For the scarce resources employed within the welfare state apparatus as a whole do all have alternative possible uses, both within and outside that apparatus. And, just as the vast resources available in the NHS might be deployed in all manner of alternative ways in order to produce all manner of different quantities of the very various goods that organization is in business to produce, so might the resources available in other parts of the UK welfare state apparatus be deployed in many different ways in order to produce different quantities of the very different but maybe almost equally various goods those other parts have been established and are maintained to produce. Economic analysis can be and sometimes is being employed to make such allocative decisions more rational in terms of the ends chosen by the deciders, just as in the Second World War economists in UK Operational Research organizations helped to guide military commanders to allocative decisions making for a speedier and less costly victory.

A First Application of the Three Principles

Now that those three fundamental and scarcely contestable principles have been firmly established it is time to begin to apply them to the workings of particular parts of the apparatus of particular welfare states. Since the universal and systematic application of these principles to the workings of welfare states both by those working within the apparatus of those welfare states and by their external critics would, hopefully, ensure that we all got better value for our tax money we might well—stealing a populist phrase from Dr. Sun Yat Sen, the founding father of the Chinese Republic—label them the Three People's Principles.

The establishment of these three principles in the previous section may well have seemed to many readers excessively longwinded. So it would have seemed to the present writer when he first tried to persuade a group of present and future public sector workers of the relevance of these principles to their present or future professional activities.[7] But abundant later experience has demonstrated that such people are in most cases extremely reluctant to recognize this relevance and to accept what are so often personally unwelcome consequent morals. So, in rather hopeless hopes that the contemporary morals may be more effectively insinuated by adopting an indirect approach, the state institutions of which the functionings and malfunctionings are to be examined here will be examined as they were a generation ago.

What called itself "The community mental health movement in the United States"[8] consisted in people who staffed programs launched under the Community Mental Health Centers Act of 1963.

That Act was passed in response to a Message to the Congress on "Mental health and mental retardation" from President Kennedy and dated February 5, 1963. In that Message he made it absolutely clear what good results were desired; and, in particular, that they were of a limited yet nonetheless important kind. For, demanding "a bold new approach," the President emphasized that "prevention is far more desirable for all concerned. It is far more economical and it is far more likely to be successful." Without himself actually specifying any illustrative examples, he called for "selected specific programs directed at known causes."

Most of my own limited knowledge of the programs that were in the event established under the resulting act, and all the quotations in the present section, derive from what was, after more than fifteen years, announced as the first of a series of "Annual Reviews of Community Mental Health."[9] All the contributors to that volume identified themselves as members of the movement; and all, it must be added, had very obvious and very strong personal stakes in the continuation and extension of the programs established under the Community Mental Health Centers Act of 1963. Judging by the contents of that book, and still more by what it does not contain, none of those involved in its compilation expected it to be studied by any critical outsiders.

With that *Annual*—as with Sherlock Holmes and the dog barking during the night—the most remarkable thing is what did not happen. For nowhere from beginning to end was one single reference, either direct or indirect, made to any evidence that any of these programs had actually succeeded in reducing the incidence of mental retardation or mental illness; or even in holding it down below the higher level to which it might perhaps otherwise have been expected to rise.

Had there been any such demonstrated successes, we can be sure that this book would have been full of references to them. Furthermore, everyone who had joined and was remaining in the movement with the prime intention of helping to prevent or cure such manifestly evil afflictions would now be rejoicing in the successes already achieved; while anyone proposing fresh initiatives towards similar ends would have been eager to learn and to apply the lessons to be drawn from past achievements and past failures.

The unlovely truth, however, is quite otherwise. These proud "prevention professionals," professed carers and compassionists though they be, did not even pretend to have fulfilled all or even any part of the beneficient mandate with which they were originally charged. Yet they appeared to be not a whit disturbed by what would seem to have been their expensive and total failure actually to prevent any specifiable and determinate evils. So, with some sideswipes against certain notoriously callous and uncaring conservative politicians—politicians suspected of contemplating what to these "prevention professionals" would have been cruel cuts in both their program and, indirectly, their individual budgets—some of them went on to propose, with no awkward self-questioning about past failures, to reinterpret the expressions "mental disease," "mental disorder," and "mental retardation" so as to facilitate demands for (yet more) further funding and extra staff. This and this alone, they suggested, would enable another and more ambitious kind of good to be done; albeit with equally little reason offered for believing that they would have any more success in attaining these different though no doubt equally worthy objectives.

In the perspective of the present chapter, the most revealing, as well as the most scandalous, feature of this entire *Annual* was the form taken by the solitary statement of the need for some systematic monitoring of success and failure. That need was simply stated, admitted, and thereafter consistently ignored. Except for the brief moment of illumination provided by the making and acceptance of that statement itself, all the contributors were inclined to identify (their) stated intentions with (their) actual achievements.

Because, they were apt to argue, our intentions were and are disinterested and beneficient, our actual achievements must inevitably and necessarily be all and only those goods that (we say) we intended; while anyone who questions those actual achievements, or challenges our demands for yet further tax funding to secure more of the same, is, upon that ground alone, to be utterly condemned. Such uncaring and uncompassionate persons deserve to be dismissed unheard as being nothing but extreme and therefore inconsiderable right-wingers.[10]

Nowhere in that *Annual* was there so much as a hint that the monitoring of actual success or failure is essential to the actual doing of a decent and progressively improving job. Instead, the sole reference to this task pointed in a quite different direction. For the only contributors who expressed concern about the lack of evidence to show what, if any, good these programs had actually done were apparently concerned only with their future funding. The trio in question made what had so far proved to be, from the standpoint of "the community mental health movement in the United States," the quite unwarrantably pessimistic statement: "it is our strong conviction that prevention proponents will lose the political battle for funding without good data—capable of documenting the effectiveness and social utility of prevention programs."[11]

Since President Kennedy had a mentally retarded sibling, and hence a strong personal interest in the success of the programs launched under the Community Mental Health Centers Act of 1963, he would, had he lived to win and to serve a second term as president, surely have demanded a progress report. It is easy to imagine his response to the "prevention professionals" tacit confession that they had no evidence at all of any successes!

A Second Application of the Three Principles

This second application is to social work and social work training in the UK. Most of my own, again, extremely limited, knowledge in this area derives directly or indirectly from my friends Colin Brewer and June Lait—mainly from their book *Can Social Work Survive*?[12] It is full of references to the almost universal unwillingness to monitor the results of social work. Thus, in chapter 1, "Beginnings: Social work, medicine and training until Seebohm,"[13] the authors note how "The [Seebohm] Committee mention without comment that an irritant to many doctors is a lack of interest of many workers in the social services, and even among the academics, in evaluating the results of their work." Brewer and Lait make their own parenthetical comment where the Seebohm Committee did not: "(It remains a profound irritant to the joint authors of this book.)"[14] For, if and in so far as social workers really are not interested in discovering what goods and what not-so-goods are in fact resulting from their activities, and if and in so far as they are not ever-ready to change their methods and practices in the light of discoveries of past success and failure, how can even their best friends continue to concede that they are sincerely and whole-heartedly in the business of doing good? The true moral to be drawn from such a sustained lack of interest is, surely, that social work activities of some established kind have become for these social workers both/either ends in themselves and/or means to some end other than the good of their (often conscript) clients.

There is indeed some reason to believe that the situation is frequently even worse than was suggested by that explanatory remark in the Report of the Seebohm Committee. It is not only or not merely that "many workers in the social services" show "a lack of interest" in themselves "evaluating the results of their work." What is far worse than this reluctance themselves to perform, or even to cooperate in, any assessment of results is the indifference to hostility shown towards the findings of what little competent research has so far been done by outsiders. Brewer and Lait notice, for example, the report of one most atypical social worker about the reactions of his colleagues to a lecture on the findings of such research:

> Sheldon was greatly disturbed by the ineffectiveness of social work which the study revealed. But he goes on to say: "I was much more worried (and still am) by the complacent smiles of colleagues all around me." He categorizes the typical response among social workers to demonstrations of their ineffectiveness as: "let's pretend nothing of importance has happened."[15]

Next, consider one or two of the accounts provided by leading figures in the world of social work of the sort of goods that everyone in that world, supposedly, is striving to do. These accounts are uniformly vague, abstract, and pretentious. None of them provides any useful clues to the solution of the problems of determining whether all tasks are being performed well or badly; or, indeed, at all. It must, therefore, be impossible to design a course of study to qualify people to perform these important, supposedly supremely skilled, yet altogether indeterminate tasks. Nevertheless, to the surprise of none of those who have spent their working lives in the university world, the manifest impossibility of providing a satisfactory course of training for such a form of employment has not prevented heads of departments eager to expand the scope of their responsibilities from volunteering to provide courses to meet this impossible demand.[16] Nor has this impossibility restrained those passing the resulting courses from asking and receiving enhanced professional salaries for exercising the subtle skills that, it is alleged, they must have acquired thereby.

Our first authoritative statement of what it is that social workers are supposed to be doing was provided by the pronouncement issued to the Mackintosh Committee[17] by Dame Eileen Younghusband. Once described by the now long since defunct weekly journal *New*

Society as "The Grand Dame of social work," she ruled that:

> The social worker is concerned with remedying certain deficiencies which may exist in the relation between the individual and his environment, and for this purpose is concerned with the total individual in relation to the whole of his environment, in so far as this is relevant to righting such deficiencies.[18]

Gouts of similarly lordly and ethereal guff spurt out all over in papers issued by the Central Council for Education and Training in Social Work: "social workers have a responsibility to individualize and personalize their clients"; their primary tasks are "communication, assessment and organizing change through the disciplined use of self"; and "in the last analysis social work is concerned with greater personal and social fulfilment in any one generation... We have to examine carefully, however, what we mean by 'fulfilment'—not all human potentials are desirable."[19]

We must not, however, allow ourselves to be so overcome by the revelatory impact of that final finding as to fail to attend to the British Association of Social Workers Discussion Paper No. 3, "The Inalienable Element in Social Work," issued over the signature of the immediate past chairman in March 1973. "The need to spell out what is the core or essence of social work," she writes, "has been around for some time." This need, we are told, was most happily met "in glorious sunshine on the sea-front at Eastbourne." To guide these philosophical investigations a Working Party explained that it had "sought to identify the quintessence of social work," but that in so doing it had deliberately not attended to "what social workers do, because this varies with the agency and with the worker."[20]

These proceedings were not only absurd but also harmful. They were absurd because there simply is no Platonic idea of Social Work "laid up in Heaven," no real essence of social work constituted by God's blueprints for that activity. How could there be since the expression "social work" was first introduced in the twentieth century, and by ordinary mortal beings, in order to refer collectively to a job lot of activities, many rather humble but some very worthy, a job lot that may well have nothing more in common than a Wittgensteinian "family resemblance"?

The same proceedings were at least potentially harmful, inasmuch as they must have tended to encourage trained social workers to believe that they must, as the result of that training, possess esoteric and precious skills, skills proportionate to the length of training and to their professional pay and status. Believing this, it becomes only natural for them to want to be exercising such skills, rather than performing only those humbler tasks that may well be all that there is usefully to be done.[21]

A Third Application of the Three Principles

In both the USA and the UK, the failure to monitor and the consequences of that failure have been most remarkable in the systems of tax-funded primary and secondary education. The public school system in the USA was in 1982, of all the contemporary systems of state-funded primary and secondary education in First World countries, perhaps the least dissimilar to the maintained school system in the UK. In neither country was there then any comprehensive national system of independently assessed and criteria—as opposed to norm-referenced—school-leaving examinations.

A system of examinations is characterized as independent in as much as the examiners are not influenced in their verdicts on the work examined by those who have had any share in the production of that work—above all the pupils themselves or their teachers. In norm-referenced examinations the examiners aim to award the same grades to roughly the same percentages of all the candidates presenting at the same time. In criteria-referenced examinations the examiners attempt the more exacting and perhaps never perfectly attainable objective of ensuring that given levels of attainment always get the same grading.

Had there been such a system of independently assessed, criteria-related school-leaving examinations in the public school system in the USA, the performance of that system could not have been so deplorable as it was found to be when in 1982 the U.S. Commission on Excellence in Education made its report under the title *A Nation at Risk.* The crucial epitomising clause in that Report read:

> The educational foundations of our society are presently being eroded by a rising tide of mediocrity that threatens our very future as a nation and as a people... If an unfriendly foreign power had attempted to impose on America the mediocre educational performance that exists today, we might well have viewed it as an act of war. As it stands, we have allowed this to happen to ourselves.

There has in the UK never been a national commission to produce a comparable report. But a very good reason to suspect that the

UK-maintained school system was at that time in a similarly disastrous condition was provided by Lord Joseph in the House of Lords' debate about the Bill that was to become the 1988 Education Reform Act (ERA). Before his elevation into the House of Lords, Sir Keith Joseph had served as minister of state in the Department of Education and Science (DES) from September 1981 until May 1986. His experienced and considered judgement was that the organization and performance of the British-maintained school system at that time constituted "a national catastrophe."[22]

Margaret Thatcher and her main political friend and ally, Sir Keith Joseph, recognized from the beginning of the first Thatcher administration the need to radically reform the UK-maintained school system. But at that time other needs were even more urgent.[23] Unfortunately, in his own years as minister of state in the DES Sir Keith Joseph failed to win the support of his Cabinet colleagues for the introduction of a tax-funded educational voucher scheme.[24]

Mark Carlisle, however, his immediate predecessor at the DES, introduced the Bill that became the 1980 Education Act. It was the "total opposition" of the National Union of Teachers (NUT), the biggest of the British teachers' unions, to one particular clause in this Bill that—to anyone aware of the logically necessary relations between sincerity of purpose, rationality, and the monitoring of success or failure in the achievement of the purposes professed—made it manifest that the British-maintained school system must have been at that time in acute need of radical reform.

For the clause to which the NUT declared its "total opposition," but which in due course did become law, required that all state-maintained schools should publish any results obtained by any of their pupils in independently assessed and (in fact at that time always) criteria-referenced examinations. In 1980 the writers of editorials and the education correspondents were all so familiar with and so uncritical about the lack of any school-leaving examinations in the state-maintained school system that it was left to one or two writers of letters to the editor to point out that not even the president of the National Union of Mineworkers, at that time by the far most powerful of all the manual workers' unions, would have had the effrontery to declare his union's "total opposition" to the publication of output statistics by the National Coal Board, the management of the then-nationalized coal industry.

One consequence of the passing of the ERA and of two or three further amending and extending Acts is that pupils in the British-state maintained school system are now subjected to frequent, perhaps excessively frequent, internal and external examinations. Thanks to these examinations, and especially to those at the primary level, it has become beyond reasonable dispute that many of those teaching in the teacher training institutions have been, and some still are, teaching, and commending as "progressive," methods of teaching—and in particular of teaching reading—demonstrably inferior to the methods they themselves despise and dismiss as old-fashioned.

The insincerity of educational purpose shown by the teachers' union objecting to the monitoring of the effectiveness of the teaching done by its members is paralleled by the insincerity of teaching purpose of these misteachers of future teachers who do not monitor the effectiveness of the teaching methods they urge pupil teachers to adopt—or rather, perhaps even worse, who ignore all evidence of the ineffectiveness of these methods when such evidence is produced by other people.

For information about the lamentable performance of the British state-maintained school system over the last fifty years see John Marks 2000. For British attempts to undo some of the ill effects of "progressive" misteaching in teacher training institutions see Jennifer Chew 1996, Turner and Burkard 1996, and John Marks 1996. For the USA, by far the best source is Jeanne S. Chall 2000. She provided both a brilliant analysis of what research tells us about effective and ineffective teaching and a mournful reflection on why there is so much of the latter.

After decades of research, Chall, who died in 1999, posed a question that should chill the blood of every policymaker: "Why were the same reforms proposed again and again, under new labels, with little recognition that they were similar to practices or policies that had failed in the past?" The victims of educational malpractice are real and numerous. Behind grim statistics like "70% of inner-city 4th graders read below grade level" are yet grimmer consequences, like a burgeoning prison population made up mostly of men whose mathematical- and verbal-literacy skills are of the eighth grade level or below.

Chall was perhaps best known for her definitive studies of reading instruction. This research demonstrated the effectiveness of phonics—teaching the relationship between letters and sounds and the ability to "decode" unfamiliar words into their correct sounds. The "whole language" reading method that Chall criticized attempts to teach sight recognition of whole words and sentences at the earliest stages of reading. Despite the evidence of its failure, whole language has enjoyed remarkable longevity. And this is precisely Chall's point: whole language has been around since the 1920s, but its advocates in the 1980s and 1990s never referred to the decades-old body of evidence warning against it. Even now we have still not seen the end of such stubborn bigotry—bigotry under the pretentious misdescription of "progressivism."

Notes

1. The nature of what is so commonly called "public money" would be brought home more vividly to one and all if only the expression "tax money" were to be systematically substituted for the expression "public money."
2. Anderson, Digby, Lait, June and Marsland, David, *Breaking the Spell of the Welfare State*, pp. 27-8 (emphases original).
3. Carroll, Lewis, 1939, pp. 677-730.
4. I have not just imagined such pretentious silliness. For in a university Senate of which I was myself a member, enquiries about the cost-effectiveness of some current educational policies were met with supercilious donnish apothegms concerning "certain prominent persons who know the cost of everything and the value of nothing."
5. By "Europe," I mean here and always geographical or merely Continental Europe, and most emphatically not the European Union (EU). Supporters of that project for the construction of a centralized superstate to rival the USA, unable directly and honestly to meet the arguments of their UK opponents, exploit this calculated ambiguity in order to denounce us as xenophobic bigots.
6. See the classical essay on "The Nature and Significance of Economic Science" in Robbins 1932.
7. It was to a group of teachers and future teachers in a College of Education. I was introduced as a specimen of that rare and exotic species, a right-wing professor. I succeeded in persuading only a small and somewhat reticent minority of my audience that anyone sincerely concerned to teach anything needs some form of—preferably independent—testing of their success or failure in this endeavour.
8. Price, R. H. et al., 1980, p. 7. This book is much more fully discussed in my article "The spending cure" in *Policy Review* for Winter 1982, pp. 178-84.
9. Price et al. 1980.
10. For a more remarkable example of such a dismissal of weighty evidence purely on partisan political grounds, see "What is to be Done?" in chapter 3, above.
11. Price et al. 1980, p. 288.
12. Brewer and Lait 1980.
13. The 1968 recommendations of the Seebohm Committee led to the passing of the Social Services Act 1970, under which local authorities were required to create social services departments to undertake the functions previously performed by children's, welfare and public health departments.

14. Brewer and Lait 1980, p. 24.
15. Ibid., p. 184.
16. I will here refrain from naming the institution in which, during a Senate debate about difficulties arising from the introduction of a bachelor of education degree course, the admissions tutor remarked: "We have made our B.Ed., and now we must lie about it."
17. Reporting in 1951 this was a Committee on Social Workers in the Mental Health Services.
18. Quoted by Brewer and Lait 1980, p. 29.
19. Quoted ibid., p. 31.
20. These BASW papers were reprinted in *Social Work Today*, Vol. 4, No. 1 (April 5, 1973). There was a regrettably gentle and conciliatory philosophical comment in Vol. 4, No. 7 (June 28, 1973).
21. Brewer and Lait presented a deal of evidence that this belief, and the consequent elevated aspirations, were widespread in the social work world.
22. House of Lords, *Hansard* for April 18, 1988, column 1263. For an instructive comparison between the U.S. and the UK systems at that time and the contemporary Japanese system, see Lynn, Richard, 1988.
23. For what these needs were see Hoskyns 2000.
24. In 1981, in response to a request from the minister, the DES put out a paper entitled simply *Education Vouchers*. This was clearly intended to kill the idea. Showing no knowledge of any of the abundant previous literature published mainly but not exclusively by the Institute of Economic Affairs, this paper raised without attempting to meet the objections already disposed of in that literature. The only extensive published criticism of that departmental paper was "Vouchers: A reply to the DES" (Flew 1982). The present writer will gladly send a photocopy of this document to anyone proposing to write a history of the voucher ideal and attempts to realize it.

7

Selfishness, Exploitation, and the Profit Motive

Besides, there is nothing so plain boring as the constant repetition of assertions that are not true, and sometimes not even faintly sensible; if we can reduce this a bit, it will be all to the good.—J. L. Austin, Sense and Sensibilia *(p. 62)*

There can be few more compelling examples of the sort of thing that the implacable Professor J. L. Austin hoped to reduce than the constantly reiterated assertion that, because they are supposedly driven by the profit motive, competitive capitalist economies must be—as compared with the socialist command alternative—peculiarly and intrinsically selfish.

Thus R H. Tawney, in his first prophetic book *The Acquisitive Society* (1921), to go no further back, excoriated a "system in which industry is carried on, not as a profession serving the public, but for the advantage of shareholders."[1] He therefore wanted "to release those who do constructive work...to apply their energies to the true purpose of industry, which is the provision of service."[2] He reflected with satisfaction, "Over a considerable field of industry, the Cooperative Movement has already substituted the motive of communal service for that of profit."[3]

A few years later, these thoughts were echoed by the then-once and future British prime minister Ramsay MacDonald: to transform "capitalism into socialism...industry must be converted from a sordid struggle for gain into a cooperative undertaking, carried on for the service of the community and amenable to its control."[4] Much later still, a few months before his death in 1955, Albert Einstein was quoted in the *Socialist International Review* as saying: "The economic anarchy of capitalist society...is the main cause of our evils. Production is carried on for profit, not for use." And so it went on, it seemed without end.

Thus, in the summer of 1972, under the headline "Waiting for a sign from the Egoists," the *Times* of London reported that Archbishop Camara of Recife, Brazil had asked a meeting of members of both Houses of Parliament in London, "Why do you not help to lay bare the serious distortions of socialism such as they exist in Russia and China? And why do you not denounce, once and for all, the intrinsic selfishness and callousness of capitalism?" As recently as 1989 Professor Raymond Plant—notwithstanding that he was at that time often credited with having striven valiantly and with rare persistence to come to terms with the by then no longer deniable failures of "actually existing socialism"—admitted only most grudgingly that "There *may* well be a place for markets in a humane society" (emphasis added), while nevertheless strongly insisting that these must be tightly confined "because they encourage some forms of behavior rather than others, viz. egoism over altruism, and rational calculation of advantage over trust."[5]

Self-Interest and Selfishness

To the archbishop's second question, the best first reply is another question: "Why is it that we never hear of the rent motive or the wages motive?" Perhaps at least the classical distinction between profit and rent is obsolete. But if it is proper to speak of a profit motive, it should be equally proper to speak of a wages motive. By parity of reasoning we shall then also have to admit into our economic psychology the fixed-interest motive, the top-price motive, the best-buy motive, and many more. And of course, if it is proper to argue that those who are paid wages must be moved by the wages motive, then it has to be not merely proper but positively refined to say that those whose wages are paid at longer intervals and are called a salary, or even compensation, are moved by, respectively, the salary motive and the compensation motive.[6]

The purpose of putting this immediate counter-question is to provoke two relevant thoughts. The first of these is that it is misguided to insist on applying to psychology a system of categories originally developed in, and appropriate to, economics. To insist on doing this is rather like postulating a set of chess motives, distinguished one from another by reference to those similarities and differences that have been found relevant to the interests and purposes of chess theoreticians, and then labeling these factitious postulations with expressions drawn from the technical vocabulary of chess—the knight's move motive, the fool's mate motive, the queening motive, and so on.

It is, surely, a venial indulgence to quote here a high classical example of such a misguided introduction of economic concepts into psychology. In *A Treatise of Human Nature*, David Hume contrived to discover that "a man, who desires a thousand pounds, has in reality a thousand or more desires, which uniting together, seem to make only one passion: tho' the composition evidently betrays itself upon every alteration of the object, by the preference he gives to the larger number, if superior only by an unite."[7] This exercise in truly heroic theorizing was presumably one of the many reasons why Hume was later to disown the *Treatise*, describing it as "that juvenile work, which the author never acknowledged..."

The second thought that should be provoked by that immediate counter-question to Archbishop Camara's question is, if you are going thus to introduce any member of some set of distinctively economic or distinctively chess concepts into your psychology, then it is altogether arbitrary to introduce one only without the others—to speak of the knight's move motive without the queening motive, for instance, or of the profit motive without the wages motive.

A second possible line of response to the challenge presented here by Archbishop Camara is to insist that no one has any business simply to assume that the desire to make a (private) profit is always and necessarily selfish and discreditable, notwithstanding that the corresponding desires to obtain a wage or a salary or a retirement income are, apparently, not.

It is, no doubt, true that all these various desires are interested in the sense that those who are guided by them are, in the immortal words of Damon Runyon, the Balzac of Broadway, "doing the best they can."[8] But precisely because this does not apply equally to all, we can find no ground here for condemning one and not the others.

This neglected fact is awkward for the denouncers. For no one, surely, is so starry-eyed as to believe that any kind of economic organization can dispense with all such interested motives. "Every economic system devised for ordinary human beings," we may read even in a tract otherwise devoutly socialist, "must have self-interest as its driving force."[9] If, therefore, one economic system is upon this particular ground to be condemned as "intrinsically selfish and heartless," then, by the same token, all economic systems must be condemned in the same terms. Yet that, of course, was not what was wanted by those who thus denounced capitalism root and branch while tolerantly discounting, as merely remediable "distortions of the economic system" whatever faults they could, however reluctantly, bring themselves to recognize in the countries that were at that time fully socialist.

There is a further and fundamental mistake here, and one that surely should never have been made by anyone with pretensions to being a moral and spiritual guide. For although all selfish actions are, necessarily, self-interested, only some interested actions are also selfish. To say that a piece of conduct was selfish is to say more than that it was interested. Selfishness is always and necessarily out of order. Interestedness is not, and scarcely could be.

For example: When two healthy children eagerly eat their dinners it would presumably be correct to say that each is pursuing his or her own interest. No doubt economists would describe them, if any choices were involved, as in this way maximizing their utilities. Yet this is no sufficient reason to reproach them. Time for that after brother has grabbed and eaten his sister's dinner as well as his own; or perhaps in some less flagrant way refused to consider others and to respect their proper claims. Even when my success can be won only at the expense of the failure of others, it would be absurd to insist that it is always and necessarily selfish for me to pursue my own interests. For is anyone prepared to say that all rival candidates competing for some coveted position are culpably selfish in not withdrawing in order to clear the way for the others?

The upshot, therefore, is that it will not wash to dismiss any one economic system as "intrinsically selfish and heartless" simply because that system depends upon and engages interested motives or even simply because it allows or encourages people to pursue their own interests in certain situations of zero-sum conflict. If there is to be something peculiarly obnoxious about wanting to make a (private) profit, then it will have to be something about making a (private) profit as such. For it would be preposterous to maintain: either that our desires to acquire economic goods for ourselves are as such improperly selfish; or that our competing to acquire scarce economic goods for ourselves in situations of zero-sum conflict is always improperly selfish.

An Aristotelian Interlude

That it is indeed essentially scandalous to make a profit and hence somewhat scandalous to wish to do so is an idea as old as the classical Greek philosophers. Consider what was said by the one who has had and who, albeit mainly through Aquinas and Hegel, has continued to have the greatest influence. Paradoxically, the economic thought of Artistotle is to be found in his *Politics*.[10] One of its characteristics was that he accepted as normative whatever he believed to be, as it were, the intentions of Nature.[11] For those inclined to follow this lead, it should be salutary to discover where it took Artistotle:

> Now if Nature makes nothing purposeless or in vain, all animals must have been made by nature for the sake of men. It also follows that the art of war is in some sense a natural mode of acquisition. Hunting is a part of that art; and hunting ought to be practised, not only against wild animals, but also against those human beings who are intended by nature to be ruled by others and refuse to obey that intention. War of this kind is naturally just.[12]

No one after reading this will be surprised to find that the universal provider envisioned by Aristotle was Nature, and not, as it would be today, the State. His position is thus oddly reminiscent of that of those contemporaries, both clerical and lay, who assume that all wealth, in the form of immediately marketable goods and services, was directly created by nature and is therefore available, free of any legitimate prior proprietorial claims, for radical redistribution by the State in accordance with the putative principles of "social" justice.[13] Aristotle went on to say:

> On a general view, as we have already noticed, a supply of property should be ready to hand. It is the business of Nature to furnish subsistence for every being brought into the world; and this is shown by the fact that the offspring of animals always gets nourishment from the residuum of the matter that gives it its birth.[14]

Aristotle thus thought that the world owes us a living or—borrowing Robert Nozick's Biblical analogy—that all wealth drops like "manna from heaven." Aristotle, consequently, emphasized acquisition rather than production:

> The natural form, therefore, of the art of acquisition is always, and in all cases, acquisition from fruits and animals. That art...has two forms: one which is connected with...trade, and another which is connected with the management of the household. Of these two forms, the latter is necessary and laudable; the former is a method of exchange which is justly censored, because the gain in which it results is not naturally made, but is made at the expense of other men.[15]

Aristotle's contention here was that any such exchange, any trade, is essentially exploitative. For he believed that the acquisitions of any trader, must necessarily be made at the expense of that trader's trading partner, whereas the only creditable acquisitions are those achieved direct from non-human nature. Shorn of these notions of what is and is not in accord with the intentions of Nature, Aristotle's was the same thesis, and the same misconception, as can be found in John Ruskin's *Unto This Last*. It was that fiercely anti-capitalist work that greatly influenced Mahatma Gandhi and many of the founding fathers of the British Labour Party. In it Ruskin insisted that "Whenever material gain follows exchange, for every plus there is a precisely equal minus."[16]

This win-lose viewpoint had for centuries been, and at least until the collapse of the Soviet empire remained, a popular misconception, especially in the form referring particularly to all trade in labor (power). For instance, an author who revealed no other Marxist cloven hoof tossed off, as if it were the most uncontentious of truisms, the remark that "the mystique of capitalism...disguises the transfer of benefits from worker to employer under the form of an equal exchange of values, through the device of a free contract of employment."[17]

The seminal mistake here provides an always welcome occasion to quote a poet-scholar's rebuke to a rival scholar's lapse: "Three minutes' thought would suffice to find this out; but thought is irksome and three minutes is a long time."[18] The crux is that trade is a reciprocal relationship. If I am trading with you, it follows necessarily that you are trading with me. Trade is also, for both parties, necessarily voluntary. Nothing that you may succeed in seizing from me by force can, by that token, have been acquired or relinquished in trade. If any possible advantage of trade to the traders could be gained only at the expense of some corresponding disadvantage to trading partners, it would appear that in any commercial exchange at least one party must be a fool, a masochist, or a gambler.

But, as all must recognize when not either by theory or by passion distracted, the truth is that sellers sell because, in their actual situations, they would rather receive the price than retain the goods while buyers buy because, in their actual situations, they would rather pay the price than be without the goods. Ruskin was therefore wrong. It is of the essence of trade not that any advantage for one party can be achieved only at the expense of the other but that no deal is made at all unless both parties believe, whether rightly or wrongly, that they stand to gain thereby; or unless at least both prefer the deal actually made to any available alternative deal or to no deal at all.

Certainly one of the trading partners, or even both, may be mistaken or in some other way misguided in the decision to deal. Certainly too the actual situation of either party, the situation in which it seems better to make the deal than not, may be in many ways unfair or unfortunate. But all this is contingent and hence irrelevant to the present question, which is: "What is and is not essential to the very idea of trade?" One temptation to conclude that trade necessarily involves a zero-sum confrontation lies in the fact that both buyers and sellers would often, if they had to, pay more or accept less than they do. Obviously, it is in such a situation possible to regard either the more that might have been gotten or the less that might have been given as an advantage forfeited by one trading partner to the other. While this may often be the case, certainly it is not so always. Both buyer and seller may be, and I imagine typically are, simultaneously in similar situations with regard to such possible but unachieved advantages. It cannot be correct to infer, as a general conclusion, that all the gains of trade must always be achieved by one trading partner at the expense of the other.

Another less intellectual but in practice more powerful temptation lies in the unappealing human inclination rather to attend with eager jealousy to the gains of others than to find a modest contentment in one's own, to forget that the deal was to your advantage in order to resent that it was also to his. Surely he would not, as you so ungraciously insist, "have made his profits out of you" had it not also been the case that you saw some advantage to yourself in your dealings with him? Yet how true it is that:

> Few men can be persuaded that they get too much by those they sell to, how extraordinary soever their gains are; when at the same time there is hardly a profit so inconsiderable, but they'll grudge it to those they buy from.[19]

Aristotle's next contribution, equally unfortunate, has been equally important. The third of the three passages just quoted from the *Politics* continues:

> The trade of the usurer is hated most, and with reason... Currency came into existence merely as a means of exchange; usury tries to make it increase. This is the reason why

> interest is called by the word we commonly use [namely, "tokos," which was Classical Greek for "offspring"]; for as the offspring resembles its parent, so the interest bred by money is like the principal which breeds it, and it may be called "currency the son of currency." Hence we can understand why, of all modes of acquisition, usury is the most unnatural.[20]

"Usury" is now, thanks first to Aristotle and still more to his medieval successors, such a bad word that we may at first fail to realize to what he is objecting. It was not only to those very high rates of fixed interest that would nowadays be condemned as usurious. Nor even was it only to all fixed interest as such. It was that which was the prime target of those medieval successors. No, Aristotle's objection here was to any money return upon any money investment. It was, he thought, against nature for money to breed money. The moment Aristotle's point is clearly appreciated, it becomes obvious that both his objection and his supporting reason were superstitious and muddled. For a sum of money is the financial equivalent of any of the goods or collections of goods that it might buy. There can, therefore, be nothing obnoxiously unnatural about receiving a money return upon an investment in money, unless it would be equally obnoxious and unnatural to ask for some return either in money or in kind for the use of the goods themselves.

Three corollaries may be drawn from this account of the essential nature of money—corollaries the drawing of which makes these further references to Aristotle of more than merely antiquarian interest. First, it has to be entirely unilluminating psychologically to speak of any money motive and, by the same token, still more unilluminating to try to develop a complete economic psychology upon a basis of a series of economic distinctions between various mercenary motives. For, that someone wants to make a profit or earn a wage tells us nothing of what he wants the money for. Almost any desire can take the form of a desire for money. It is obvious that this is a necessary consequence of the essential nature of money as a conventional instrument of exchange. Aristotle himself elsewhere makes this point about the nature of money. Nevertheless, as we have just seen, he fails to appreciate its present application.

The second corollary is that it has to be wrong to hope that the abolition of money or even a reduction of the range of desired goods that money can buy might by itself reduce greed and competition. Certainly it is tautologically true that the profit motive, the fixed-interest motive, the wages motive, and all the other factitious economic motives so far listed or suggested are mercenary. All, that is, may be defined in terms of the acquisition of money. It might therefore seem that to totally abolish money or reduce its importance as a means of acquisition must be to abolish or at least weaken all mercenary motives.

In an appropriately empty sense no doubt this is true. Yet, unless these changes happened to be accompanied by something quite different—an enormous transformation of present human nature—people would presumably continue to pursue, and to compete for, whatever it was that they had always wanted but that money could not now buy. In a word: if cars are not on sale for money but are available as a perquisite of public office, then this will by itself tend only to intensify the competition for such privileged official positions—a result long familiar to those who studied the actual operation of Soviet-type economies (STEs) in Eastern Europe and elsewhere. For, by itself, and short of the aforesaid total transformation of human nature, the abolition of money could not and would not so much as begin to make us either less materialistic or less competitive.

The third corollary is that money, and the extension of the range of goods and services that money can buy, are sovereign instruments of choice. If rewards are offered not in money but in kind, then recipients are precisely not allowed to choose. Whoever fixes the rewards then determines not only their sizes but also what they are all to be. And if and to the extent that, for instance, health, education, and welfare services are monopolistically provided by a state, its citizens will be deprived of any direct and individual choice of what quantity and quality of such services they wish to use.[21] Even more important, they will be deprived of all the benefits that competition between rival suppliers might and surely would bring.

Wants or Needs, Choice or Command

In *A Critique of the Gotha Programme*, Karl Marx famously proclaimed a distributive ideal that many have found appealing: "From each according to their abilities, to each according to their needs." Few, it seems, have caught the sinister overtones both of authoritarianism and of austerity in that slogan. (Perhaps these were missed even by Marx himself.) But necessities are most typically and naturally contrasted with luxurious superfluities; and although we are all of us the best experts about our own *wants*, it is others who are so eager to tell us that what we *really need* is altogether different, and usually, at least to us, more or less disagreeable.[22] How too, save by compulsion, is it to be ensured that after all individual incentives have been eliminated all will labor at their prescribed tasks to the limits of their abilities?

Aristotle maintained, as we have just been reminded, that trading exchanges are always and essentially exploitative. In the same passage he made a precarious distinction between two forms of the art of acquisition, acquisition for household use and acquisition for financial gain. This distinction is precarious because producers for a market cannot expect to make any profits save in so far as there are customers able and willing to purchase their products. Presumably such customers propose to use whatever they buy in some way, judging that that employment is necessary in order to satisfy one or more of their own wants.

The true antithesis here is, of course, that between a market and a command economy. In the former, producers produce what they believe they can find people able and willing to buy. In the latter, what is produced is whatever the actual power elites both within and above the organizations of production order to be produced. That is likely to be some synthesis of what the members of those elites want for themselves and what they are content that the lower orders should have. From the foundation of the Centre for Research into Communist Economies[23] in 1983, more information than ever before began to become available about the preference structure of the power elite in the USSR. What—to borrow General Lee's phrase for describing Union armies—"those people" wanted most for themselves was, of course, in order to maintain and to extend their power, enormous and efficiently equipped military and police forces. What they considered to be sufficient to meet the needs of the rest of the Soviet people was, by the standards of contemporary democratic capitalism, simply wretched.[24]

There is a fatal flaw in the assertion that, because supposedly they are driven by the profit motive, competitive capitalist economies must be, compared with the socialist command alternative, peculiarly and intrinsically selfish. It is that it depends upon an invalid form of inference. This invalid form of inference proceeds from propositions about the purposes attributed to institutions and to the people establishing these institutions to conclusions about the actual operative motives of the future managers and employees of these institutions.

There is no disputing that the management of any firm that wants to stay in business and has no access to any open-ended subsidy has to pay constant attention to the bottom line. Yet, from this fundamental and undisputed fact about private business we are most emphatically not entitled to infer that obtaining and maximizing profits is necessarily and throughout all working hours the exclusive and overriding concern of the management, much less that that must be the predominant or indeed any very noticeable concern of all the employees.

To keep profitable is in the long run a necessary condition of staying in business. But that is by no means a sufficient or indeed any sort of good reason for insisting that the only motive that anyone can or does have for going into or staying in business is to obtain for themselves the maximum possible profit. Furthermore, not only is the argument to this cynical conclusion invalid but the conclusion itself is also in fact false, if only because very few of us ever manage to be so utterly single-minded about anything. Many, too, have had occasion to rue the fact that such a single-minded profit orientation was far from characteristic of some firms in which they themselves had invested, while everyone in everyday commercial dealings must surely have enjoyed at least some friendly and considerate treatment that quite obviously was not motivated by a pure and exclusive pursuit of financial gain.

Nor, of course, is the fact that some productive enterprise is a state-owned monopoly or that some other organization was specifically established by the state in order to serve the public interest any guarantee that those employed in their operation will either already be or by these facts be encouraged to become, not only more altruistic and less egoistic, but also more trusting and less given to any "rational calculation of advantage" than the rest of us. If Professor Plant does still believe that it is a valid guarantee, then the only remedy possible to prescribe for his misconception is a course of reading in the economics of public choice.[25]

The uncomfortable inquiry that should be pressed upon Professor Plant and upon all those others who share his intrusive interest in the motives of economic agents is simply, "Why?"—or, more aggressively, "By what right?" If people sell me satisfactory products at competitive prices, then it is surely no business of mine to pry into their motives for first making or otherwise acquiring these products and then selling them to me and to anyone else able and willing to pay the prices charged. Such intimate investigations are properly left to their chosen spiritual advisers, if any.

In general, and it is a reflection that has wide relevance, economic arrangements are best judged by results. Concentrate on the price and quality of the product. Do not officiously probe the producer's purity of heart. It is difficult to avoid diagnosing this eagerness to pursue such irrelevant and intrusive probings as springing from anything but a stubborn refusal to accept that socialism has most decisively failed the test of judgment by results, combined with a desperate hope that it might still be saved by an appeal to its supposedly altruistic intentions.

Where questions about motives are out of place, however, questions about interests may be very much to the point. For even the most minimally prudent persons must always hope, and try to ensure, that their suppliers have some material interest in supplying them to their satisfaction; and this quite irrespective of whether or not such interests provide the main or sole operative motives of the suppliers. You do not need to be the total cynic to feel anxious about the quality and reliability of supply where the suppliers have no interest in giving satisfaction and where their clients have to depend on the universal presence and strength of "the motive of communal service"—one of the goods that is notoriously almost always and everywhere scarce. Adam Smith, the author of *An Inquiry into the Nature and Causes of the Wealth of Nations*, the first and only classic of development economics, was his usual humane and realistic self when he wrote:

> It is not from the benevolence of the butcher, the brewer, or the baker that we expect our dinner, but from their regard for their own interest. We address ourselves, not to their humanity but to their self-love, and never talk to them of our own necessities but of their advantages. Nobody but a beggar chooses to depend chiefly upon the benevolence of his fellow citizens.[26]

Notes

1. *The Acquisitive Society*, p. 140.
2. Ibid., p. 150.
3. Ibid. p. 152. Tawney 1931, the enormously influential book that made so many converts to socialism—including in his youth the present writer—was not so concerned with the motives attributed to capitalists.
4. Quoted in Beer, S. H., *British Politics in the Collectivist Age* (London: Routledge, 1972), p. 136.
5. Hoover, K. and Plant, R., *Conservative Capitalism in Britain and the United States: A Critical Appraisal* (London: Routledge, 1989), p. 232.
6. The classic comment on such prissy synonyms for the monosyllabic "wages" and "pay" can be found in Bernard de Mandeville [1729] 1970, p. 66:

   And when folks understood their cant
   They changed that for "emolument";
   Unwilling to be short or plain,
   In any thing concerning gain…
7. I(iii)12:141.
8. See Runyon 1950, passim.
9. Lewis, W. A., 1949, p. 7.
10. The reason is that his *Economics* dealt with household management. For that is what that title meant in Classical Greek.
11. He might well have spoken enigmatically, like Spinoza, of "God or Nature."
12. 1256B 20-26, pp. 25-6.
13. See chapters 4, above, and 8, below.
14. Aristotle *Politics*, 1258A 33-6, p. 34.
15. Ibid., 1258A 37-1258B2, pp. 34-50.
16. Ruskin 1899, p. 131. This 1899 book consisted in a series of articles originally published in *Cornhill Magazine* considerably earlier.
17. Miller 1976, p. 204.
18. Housman 1905, p. xi.
19. Mandeville [1729] 1970, p. 113.
20. Aristotle *Politics*, 1258B 2-8, p. 35.
21. See Seldon 1977.
22. See Flew 1981, chapter 5.
23. It was, of course, founded under the auspices of the Institute of Economic Affairs in London. It has, since the collapse of most of those economies, been dissolved.
24. See, for instance, Eberstadt, Nick, 1988, Rowen, Henry and Wolf, Charles (eds.), 1990, and Roberts, Paul Craig and La Follette, Karen, 1990.
25. The two essentials for a short course are Mitchell 1980 and Tullock, Seldon, and Brady 2000. But instructive relief is available in *The Complete Yes Minister*, Lynn and Jay 1988.
26. Smith [1776] 1981, Book I, chapter 2, p. 27.

8

"Social" Justice and Private Property

I had tried to show for a large number of instances that what was claimed as demanded by "social justice" could not be justice because the underlying consideration (one could hardly call it a principle) was not capable of general application... I have now become convinced, however, that the people who habitually employ the phrase simply do not know themselves what they mean by it and just use it as an assertion that a claim is justified without giving a reason for it.
—F. A. Hayek, Preface to The Mirage of Social Justice *(1976)*

Because *A Theory of Justice*[1] by John Rawls attempted to satisfy the need for some clear formulation and persuasive rationalization of the putative principles of "social" justice, it received on its first appearance such a wide and overwhelmingly enthusiastic welcome that it at once became, and has ever since remained, the standard starting point for all subsequent discussion. For instance, immediately after its first publication, the lifelong British social democrat Stuart Hampshire wrote in a notably uncritical "Critical Notice" in the *New York Review of Books*[2]:

> I think that this book is the most substantial and interesting contribution to moral philosophy since the war, at least if one thinks only of books written in English. It is a very persuasive book, being very well argued and carefully composed.

But did that Book Deserve such Adulation?

It presents, Hampshire continued: "A noble, coherent, highly abstract picture of the fair society, as social democrats see it." The political principles that are in Europe described as social democratic have for a long time been characterised in the USA as liberal. Thus, the sometime Senator Joseph S. Clark Jr., when he was mayor of Philadelphia, described the modern "liberal" position very clearly:

> To lay ghost at the outset and to dismiss semantics, a liberal is here defined as one who believes in utilising the full force of government for the advancement of social, political, and economic justice at the municipal, state, national, and international levels... A liberal believes government is a proper tool to use in the development of a society which attempts to carry out Christian principles of conduct into practical effect.[3]

A Theory of Justice had, from the beginning, and continues to maintain, a similarly strong appeal to those Americans who see themselves as liberals and to those Europeans who see themselves as social democrats.

The first and what ought to have been the most devastating of objections to this book is that Rawls makes no attempt to justify his assumption that what he presents as social justice is indeed a kind of justice. For although he entitles his six hundred and seven-page book *A Theory of Justice* he reveals as early as page seven that his true subject "is that of social justice. For us the primary subject of justice is the basic structure of society, or more exactly, the way in which the major social institutions distribute fundamental rights and duties and determine the division of the advantages from social cooperation." To this, the most fundamental philosophical objection is that of Hayek: "to apply the term 'just' to circumstances other than human actions or the rules governing them"—such as the operation of social institutions or the behavior of some hypostatised Society—"is a category mistake,"[4] a mistake, that is, such as would be made by a person who asked for the color of a speed or the number of an aberration.

Some might dismiss such a philosophical objection as merely verbal. Certainly Rawls himself seems never to have felt the force of the warning Plato scripted his Socrates to utter in the last words of Book I of *The Republic*[5]: "For if I do not know what justice is I am scarcely likely to find out whether it is an excellence and whether its possessor is happy or not happy." This is a warning to which Rawls not so much fails as refuses to attend. For he never finds room to quote, much less examine, either some variant of the traditional definition of the word "justice," or any preferred alternative. Indeed, it is only on his five hundred and seventy-ninth page that he thinks to explain, without any suggestion of apology, that he was eager "to leave questions of meaning and definition aside and get on with the task of developing a substantive theory of (*sic*) justice."[6] Rawls thus surely became the first person to present as a treatise on justice a massive volume making no reference at all to the great juridical tradition stretching back to the *Institutes* of Justinian and beyond.

Among those who have actually asked themselves the question "What is justice?" there seems, at least until comparatively recently, to have been little disagreement. The central, crucial element in all definitions has always been what Plato scripted Polemarchus to offer as his first suggestion: "to render to each his due,"[7] a phrase later translated into Latin as *suum cuique tribuere*. Ulpian prefaced this with two further clauses, making his own definition, which was followed by the *Institutes* of Justinian: *Honeste vivere, neminem laedere, suum cuique tribuere* (To live honestly, to injure no one, to render to each *suum jus* [his own]). That last Latin expression plainly is to be construed as referring not to the operation of "the major social institutions," but to the several and often very different deserts and entitlements of different individuals. We need here, however, to distinguish between the concept and conceptions of justice. For although there has apparently been little disagreement about the concept of justice, there have of course been rival conceptions both of what people's moral and legal deserts and entitlements are and of how these are properly to be determined.

At this point, if not much earlier, some might perhaps protest that all this insisting upon and drawing out the implications of the traditional definition of the word "justice" is so much verbal trifling. These protesters might be wanting us, to coin a phrase, "to leave questions of meaning and definition aside and to get on with the task of developing a substantive theory," if not of dull, old, unfashionable, without prefix or suffix justice, then of swinging, trendy, with-it social justice. But to anyone who persists in describing as just the implementation of a favored project that cannot be correctly so characterized, the proper response is to ask why, if the application of one word rather than another is really a matter of no importance, they remain resolved to employ the term "justice" instead of some newly-minted alternative.

The reason, of course, is that these protesters propose to continue behaving as if, when employed in another sense, the word "justice" would still carry the same implications as it did before it was given that new employment. But the truth is that, unless what they call social justice can be shown to be a kind of justice, as traditionally understood, those with "a passion for social justice" cannot as such be entitled either to see themselves and to be seen as legitimate occupants of the moral high ground or to draw on the forces of the state to realize what are only their purely personal and individual ideals. For, as in his other masterpiece, *The Theory of the Moral Sentiments*, Adam Smith so clearly and so unequivocally insisted:

> The man who barely abstains from violating either the person, or the state, or the reputation of his neighbours, has, surely, little positive merit. He fulfils, however, all the rules of what is peculiarly called justice, and does everything which his equals can with propriety force him to do, or which they can punish him for not doing (II [ii] 1).

Consider now the *Report* of the Commission on Social Justice established in 1992 by the then-leader of the British Labour Party, John Smith.[8] He was said in the Preface to have "allied a passion for social justice with a vision of economic renewal."[9] That Preface goes on at once to inform us that "the Commission was launched in 1992, the fiftieth anniversary of the pathbreaking Beveridge Report *Social Insurance and Allied Services*, which became the foundation of the welfare state in the UK"[10]; thus suggesting that the achievement of social justice is seen as closely if not essentially connected with the establishment and maintenance of a welfare state. The Introduction explains that:

> The values of social justice are...the equal worth of all citizens, their equal right to be able to meet their basic needs, the need to spread opportunities and life chances as widely as possible, and the requirement that we reduce and where possible eliminate unjustified inequalities.[11]

Later this statement is repeated in a somewhat fuller form. But nowhere are we told either why these values are supposed to be elements of a kind of justice or why that kind of justice requires that all inequalities be eliminated unless they can be shown to be somehow justified.

If anyone was seeking classical authority for this supposed requirement of justice, they might hope to find it in Aristotle's treatment of distributive justice, a category he was the first to introduce, in Book V of the *Nicomachean Ethics*. There Aristotle wrote: "If then the unjust is the unequal, the just is the equal—a view that commends itself to all without proof..." But Aristotle went on at once to argue that "if the persons are not equal they will not have equal shares." So Aristotle's actual conclusion was not a substantial practical prescription but a purely formal principle. It was not that equal shares for all is the imperative of justice. Rather, it was that the rules of justice, like all rules, require, not that all cases, but only that all relevantly like cases, should be treated alike.

There would thus seem to be a need in discussions of "social" justice both for a distinction introduced by William Frankena and for the term that he coined to mark it. It is one thing to *justify* something, that is, to show it to be desirable or excusable or in some other way preferable to the available alternatives, but it is quite another thing to *justicize* it, that is to show it to be not just "socially" just but plain old-fashioned, without prefix or suffix, just.[12] Hayek was however mistaken to maintain "that the people who habitually employ the phrase [social justice] just use it as an assertion that a claim is justified without giving a reason for it."[13] For anyone asserting that some policy is required by a kind of justice is in fact giving what—if but only if their assertions were true—would constitute the best of reasons.

The truth, however, is that social justice as customarily conceived is precisely not a kind of justice. On the contrary, such "social" justice essentially involves what, by the standards of the old fashioned, without prefix or suffix, sort of justice must constitute a paradigm case of flagrant injustice: the abstraction under the threat of force (the taxing away) of some of what must be defeasibly presumed to be the justly acquired income and capital of the better off in order to give it (less, of course, some often substantial service charge) to those whose previous just acquisitions or lack of just acquisitions have left them worse off.

This point, that the direct taxation of wealth and income constitutes a kind of robbery under the threat of violence, and hence that although it may be abundantly justified, it simply cannot be justicized, ought to seem obvious. But today, and to most citizens of the democratic welfare states, the making of this once obvious point is likely instead to appear perversely paradoxical, even perhaps intolerably right-wing. For we have all lived most if not all our lives in such mature welfare states. And these are states in which 40 percent and more of the GNP is spent by central and local government, states in which every perceived social evil is seen as requiring tax-funded government action, and states in which any finance minister proposing to reduce the amount taken in tax from some set[14] of citizens is said—usually accusingly—to be proposing to give that amount to members of that set rather than to allow them to retain it.

If we were still living in one of the pre-World War I democracies, in which the activities of the state were linked almost exclusively to the fulfillment of its fundamental protective functions, and in which the share of GNP spent by the state rarely, save in time of war, exceeded about 10 percent, then the financing of some of this supply of protection by direct taxation could plausibly be justified as the compulsory liquidation of debts, of payments due in return for services rendered. But this cannot of course be said of any direct taxation levied to finance redistribution. Such redistributive taxation of what we must, albeit defeasibly, presume to be the justly acquired incomes and capitals of its better off citizens is manifestly theft by the state—theft arbitrarily legitimized by that same state.

It may help to shake prejudices acquired from living in such mature welfare states, and to enable some to see that the true paradox is to describe ceasing to seize as generously donating, if we now quote some comments made in 1884 on the introduction in that year of an extremely modest income tax by sober and well-informed U.S. citizens who, up to that time, had lived all their lives under a strictly limited, classically liberal government. Commenting on this, the *New York Times* asserted that it was a "vicious, inequitable, unpopular, impolitic and socialistic act...the most unreasoning and un-American movement in the politics of the last quarter-century." And the *Chicago Tribune* added that this tax "can only be collected by prying into the private affairs of the people by arbitrary methods hateful to the citizens of the republic." In 1909, when the 16th Amendment to the Constitution, licensing the imposition of a federal income tax, was being debated, the *New York Times* criticized it, saying: "When men get into the habit of helping themselves to the property of others, they cannot easily be cured of it." History has proven that prediction correct, although the *New York Times* itself, like so many others, no longer recognizes such legalized seizures as robbery under the threat of force.

A Digression Concerning Equal Value

The Introduction to the Report of the Labour Party Commission on Social Justice informs us, as we have just seen, that one of "The values of social justice" is "the equal worth of all citizens." If anyone were to want to preserve this grotesque and perverse conclusion, s/he would have to systematically devalue every possible human characteristic, action, or achievement. For if any type or token of any of these is allowed to be preferable to any other, one could scarcely hope to show that all the actual and now admitted evaluative superiorities and inferiorities either just by chance cancel each other out, or else are so guided by Providence as to ensure that they always and reliably do.

It therefore becomes clear that the principle of "the equal worth of all citizens" is one to which its adherents are attached: not because, in the light of careful and critical consideration, it appears correct; but because, however intrinsically implausible, it seems to them either to follow from or to be presupposed by some prior, absolutely inescapable commitment.

The contexts in which some people insist upon this Principle of Equal Value are those in which others appeal to the Principle of Equal Consideration. So let us now call in evidence some famous manifesto commitments. One that is surely relevant is that essential but awkward addendum to "the Great Happiness principle" of classical Utilitarianism: "everyone to count as one and none as more than one." Then again, no historically instructed Englishman could fail to seize an occasion to quote a claim made by the russet-coated Captain Thomas Rainborough during the Putney debates of the New Model Army: "And I do believe that the poorest he that is in England hath a life to live, as much as the greatest he."

But perhaps the most familiar of all such manifesto commitments is to be found in the American Declaration of Independence: "We hold these truths to be self-evident, that all men are created equal, that they are endowed by their Creator with certain unalienable rights, that among these are Life, Liberty and the pursuit of Happiness." We shall, in the section entitled "Justice as Fairness or Justice as Justice?" be considering the justificatory rationale for these allegedly self-evident truths.

The Unargued Socialist Assumption

The fundamental principles of what Rawls calls social justice are derived from his hypothetical social contract. Although he claims that "Throughout the choice between a private-property economy and socialism is left open...,"[15] his hypothetical contracting parties who "in the original position" are to make the hypothetical social contract nevertheless have to take for granted the ultimately collective ownership of all wealth and income. "For simplicity," rather than for any more substantial reason, they are required to "assume that the chief primary goods *at the disposition of society* are rights and liberties, powers and opportunities, income and wealth."[16]

This enormous and totally unargued socialist assumption might perhaps be appropriate for people laboring to discover the proper pattern for the centrally planned and enforced distribution of all such goods in their ideal socialist state. But for someone who is supposed to be asking whether and how far actual distributions are just and, where and in so far as they are not what state-enforced (re)distributive transfers are or and would be mandated by justice, that assumption is altogether inappropriate and totally misleading. For it precisely is that all those listed "chief primary goods" already are "at the disposition of society"; that is to say that they are now freely available for redistribution at the absolute discretion of some supreme authority, altogether unhampered by any morally prior claims to possession.

The contracting parties are also conceived as operating behind a Veil of Ignorance: "...no one knows his place in society, his class position or social status; nor does he know his fortune in the distribution of natural assets and abilities, his intelligence and the like."[17] Although it is usually considered that this Veil of Ignorance is drawn in order to secure impartiality (which would make the whole exercise of comprehensive blinkering a dramatization of the colorless Humian appeal to the impartial spectator), the stated primary purpose is quite different and altogether preposterous. Thus, in explaining "The Main idea of the Theory," Rawls asserts:

> Once we decide to look for a conception of justice that nullifies the accidents of natural endowment and the contingencies of social circumstances as counters in the quest for political and economic advantage, we are led to these principles. *They express the result of leaving aside those aspects of the social world that seem arbitrary from a moral point of view.*[18]

The preposterousness is to present this as a first and necessary step towards developing of a conception of a sort of *justice*. Certainly, if all possible grounds for any differences in deserts and entitlements are thus to be dismissed as morally irrelevant, then—assuming that anyone is still to be allowed to deserve or to be entitled to anything at all—it does indeed become obvious that everyone's just deserts and entitlements must be equal. Yet it is precisely and only upon what individuals severally and individually are, on what has happened and not happened to them, and on what they have done or failed to do, that their several and often extremely unequal individual deserts and entitlements cannot but be based. It is, therefore, bizarre so superciliously to dismiss all this as irrelevant, as merely "the accidents of natural endowment and the contingencies of social circumstance."

But Rawls, although offering no substantial reason for assuming that all income and capital is collectively owned and hence remains freely available for collective (re)distribution, does offer some reasons for refusing to recognize individual deserts and entitlements. He argues against desert on two grounds: first, that our natural endowments are not themselves deserved; and, second, that, in consequence, what they make possible cannot be either itself deserved or a proper basis of desert. "Even the willingness to make an effort, to try, and so be deserving in the ordinary sense is itself dependent upon happy family and social circumstances."[19]

For Rawls, therefore, entitlements cannot be deserved. Since he sees the distribution of natural capacities as an "outcome of the natural lottery,"[20] he has apparently never even entertained the possibility of an Aristotle-type distinction between the deserved (positively good), the undeserved (positively bad), and the not-deserved (neutral). And, since he has without reference to any classical authority somehow persuaded himself that "the first principle of justice" is "one requiring equal distribution,"[21] he concludes that "undeserved inequalities call for redress; and since inequalities of birth and natural endowment are undeserved, these inequalities are to be somehow compensated for."[22]

Rawls himself provides two examples of what are in fact not-deserved entitlements, though he fails to recognize them as such. The first is what he calls the priority of liberty: "each person's equal right to the most extensive liberty compatible with a similar liberty for others."[23] These equal rights are, surely, the universal option rights eloquently proclaimed as self-evident in the American Declaration of Independence. And such rights constitute a paradigm case of justified though surely unearned and hence not-deserved entitlements. The second example in *A Theory to Justice* is the assumed collective property right of the hypothetical contractors to all wealth and income accruing, but presumably not collectively earned, within the by them temporarily forgotten territories of the state of which they are citizens. As will soon become clear, this crucial collectivist assumption cannot be reconciled with the traditional rationale for the rights proclaimed in the Declaration.

Justice as Fairness or Justice as Justice?

After the captivating frankness of the confession that we want to define "the original position so that we get the desired solution",[24] and after the hypothetical contracting parties have therefore been made to assume both that all relevant property is collectively owned and that all individual differences in social situation and personal achievement are morally irrelevant, it should come as no surprise that they cannot but "acknowledge as the first principle of justice one requiring an equal distribution. Indeed, this principle is so obvious that we would expect it to occur to anyone immediately."[25]

Granted these Rawlsian assumptions indeed it might. But, on second thoughts, it ought to occur to someone that that would be a first principle (not of justice but) of fairness in distribution (only and precisely) where no question of justice arises rather than a first principle of justice. Rawls himself offers his account of social justice as an account of (unqualified) "justice as fairness." But he gives no sign of appreciating the nature and extent of the differences between the concepts of justice and of fairness. This stubborn failure has led to some mischievous and irreverent critics of Rawls's "noble, coherent, highly abstract picture of the fair society, as social democrats see it" to suggest that the author of *A Theory of Justice* would be ideally suited to a position as general editor of a series of equally obese and misguiding studies of something as something else—works with titles such as *Marriage as Cohabitation*, *Freedom as Necessity*, and *Property as Theft*.

Many other enthusiasts for the implementation of what they call social justice have followed Rawls in choosing to adopt fundamental premises for no other or better reason than that they will yield the conclusions desired. Consider, for example, the case of the author of one of the first volumes in the then-new Library of Welfare and Philosophy. Having sketched a Rawlsian account of (social) justice as mandating a (qualified) equality of outcome he remarks that "one reason for linking equality and justice is that within the theory of justice one can then provide the necessary moral premise for adopting the principle of equal welfare as a prescriptive recommendation."[26] The properly crushing counter to such manoeuvres was provided long ago by Russell: "The method of 'postulating' what we want has many advantages; they are the same as the advantages of theft over honest toil."[27]

Enough has by now been said about the lack of warrant for making the assumptions Rawls makes in order that to "define the original position" he gets, what is for him, "the desired solution"—that "the first principle of justice" is "one requiring an equal distribution." It is time to contend that any principle derived from these assumptions is thereby disqualified from constituting a principle of justice. The reason is simple but sufficient. It is that no suggestions of just distribution can arise among a population that has no just deserts or just entitlements with respect to what is to be distributed among them.

What can, however, be derived from such assumptions is what could defeasibly be presumed to be a reasonable pattern for the distribution of some property that its owners wanted to distribute among some chosen population. Consider for instance, Isaiah Berlin's argument for a rational presumption in favor of equal distribution: "If I have a cake, and there are ten persons among whom I wish to divide it, then if I give exactly one tenth to each, this will not, at any rate automatically, call for justification; whereas if I depart from this principle of equal division I am expected to produce a special reason."[28]

But this sort of argument, which is at best directly relevant only to questions of justification in general rather than of justicization in particular, is concerned only with what would be the defeasibly rational way for someone to distribute some or all his own property that he wanted to distribute among a set of people of his own choice. Certainly it expresses a principle that "might be important if some benefactor of the human race were to wake up one morning with his pockets stuffed full of money which he wished to distribute so as to produce a maximum of enjoyment, but it has very little relation to the state of the world as we know it."[29] The trouble is that Rawls—by assuming that all the wealth and income produced and to be produced within the to them unknown territories of the state of which they are temporarily unwitting citizens is the collective property of his hypothetical contractors—is assuming that that wealth and income constitutes, as his most brilliant critic delighted to put it, "manna-from-heaven"[30]: an unearned collective windfall gain.

The most fundamental and decisive objection to the theory construction of Rawls is that it is based upon three monster, not to say monstrous, assumptions. There is, first, the socialist assumption that all "income and wealth" is "at the disposition of society." Then, second, there is the assumption that "the accidents and contingencies of social circumstances" are "from a moral point of view irrelevant."[31] Although we are never given any examples of these irrelevances they must surely include every individual's particular and different property rights. Their unstated inclusion thus provides an unstated justification for the first, socialist assumption. Third and finally there is the assumption that "since the accidents and contingencies of social circumstances" are, from a moral point of view irrelevant, we must "undertake to regard the distribution of natural abilities as a collective asset, so that the more fortunate are to benefit *only* in ways that help those who have lost out."[32]

These assumptions are said by Rawls to be necessary if he is to reach his desired conclusions about "social" justice. So let us consider another, simpler and more straightforward example of the making of the first for the same purpose. It was provided by *An Approach to Social Policy*, an official document of the National Economic and Social Council of the Republic of Ireland, drafted by D. V. Donnison and published in 1975 by the Stationery Office in Dublin. From it we discover that that Council was, by its terms of reference, required to "promote social justice," which for them apparently either involves or simply is "the fair and equitable distribution of the income and wealth of the nation."

There is here, of course, a crucial confusion. The expression "the national wealth" is a most important member of the class of what Gilbert Ryle identified as "Systematically Misleading Expressions."[33] For it misleadingly confounds the sum of the income and wealth of all the individual citizens and firms in a nation-state with the sum of the income collectively acquired and the wealth collectively owned by that state as such. Since Professor D. V. Donnison[34] has been a lifelong member of the Labour Party and was later to become a member of its above-mentioned Commission on Social Justice, we may well see the production of this document for the Republic of Ireland as a step on the road between the two understandings of the word "socialism" distinguished by Hayek in his Preface to the 1976 second edition of *The Road to Serfdom*:

> At the time I wrote socialism meant unambiguously the nationalisation of the means of production and the central economic planning which this made possible and necessary.

But in the more than thirty years since Hayek wrote that book:

> ...socialism has come to mean chiefly the extensive redistribution of incomes through taxation and the institutions of the welfare state. In the latter the effects I discuss in this book are brought about more slowly, indirectly and imperfectly. I believe that the ultimate outcome tends to be very much the same...

The Property Presuppositions of the Priority of Liberty

In from the beginning insisting upon the priority of liberty Rawls was, presumably, implicitly referring to the first words of the second paragraph of the Declaration of Independence: "We hold these Truths to be self-evident, that all Men are created equal, that they are endowed by their Creator with certain unalienable Rights, that among these are Life, Liberty and the Pursuit of Happiness..." To understand why "these Truths" appeared self-evident to the Signers it is necessary to pay some attention to the political philosophy of John Locke, something with which young Mr. Jefferson—to whom, thanks to his "peculiar felicity of expression," the drafting job had been given—was certainly familiar.

The political philosophy of John Locke was expressed in his *Two Treatises of Government*, first published in 1690, almost exactly a century before the adoption of the American Constitution. Although first published after the British Glorious Revolution, which established peacefully a new constitutional settlement under the Dutch-born King William, it was largely written earlier and in a period in which Locke was himself involved in assisting his patient and patron, the first Earl of Shaftesbury, in the political struggles that eventually achieved that new constitutional settlement.

The first of these *Two Treatises* was in its day crucially important. Nowadays it is read only by extremely conscientious or somewhat eccentric scholars. In it Locke refuted the established doctrine of the Divine Right of Kings. That was the doctrine that all legitimate kings are and must be endowed with their sovereign powers and duties by God. The first chapter of the *Second Treatise* reviews the conclusion of the *First Treatise*. Then, in the first two paragraphs of the second chapter, Locke introduces his three key ideas: first, the idea of a State of Nature; second, the idea of a reciprocal equality of individual freedom rights and individual freedom duties; and, third, the idea of these reciprocal freedom rights and freedom duties as arising from and conditioned by the Law of Nature. The first of these two paragraphs reads:

> To understand Political Power right, and derive it from its Original, we must consider what State all men are naturally in, and that is, a *State of perfect Freedom* to order their Actions, and Dispose of their Possessions, and Persons as they think fit, within the bounds of the Law of Nature, without asking leave, or depending upon the Will of any other Man.

The second of these two complementary paragraphs reads:

> A *State* also of *Equality*, wherein all the Power and Jurisdiction is reciprocal, no one having more than another: there being nothing more evident, than that Creatures of the same species and rank promiscuously born to all the same advantages of Nature, and the use of the same facilities, should also be equal one amongst another without Subordination or Subjection, unless the Lord and Master of them all, should by any manifest Declaration of his Will set one above another, and confer on him by an evident and clear appointment an undoubted right of Dominion and Sovereignty.

The first common confusion here that needs to be dispelled concerns the idea of a State of Nature. This idea should be recognized as the fertile theoretical fiction it is rather than misinterpreted as a misguided exercise in historical speculation. This theoretical fiction of an original state of nature was intended to reveal how it would be reasonable for human beings as essentially rational animals to behave under the conditions stipulated. Nor must we allow ourselves to be misled here by Bertrand Russell's deriding of Aristotle's definition of man as "the rational animal," for Aristotle, as, of course, Russell knew perfectly well, was, in offering this famous definition, not foolishly intending to commend our species as one consisting entirely of beings always, in both their thought and behavior, perfectly rational as opposed to irrational. Instead, Aristotle wanted to distinguish it as one uniquely consisting of creatures *capable* of both rational thought and rational behavior whatever the nature of their actual performance.

Some may at this point recall that, during the Senate hearings on the nomination of Clarence Thomas to the Supreme Court, one senator, whom it is charitable to refrain from naming here, objected that that nominee's belief in the subsistence of a normative Law of Nature disqualified him for that proposed appointment. Since it is difficult to believe that that, or any other senator, was unaware that the very first sentence of the Declaration of Independence contains the now apparently unacceptable phrase "the Laws of Nature and of

Nature's God," it is better to interpret his objection as rising from a well-justified fear that Clarence Thomas would, if appointed, be so conservative as to have doubts about the constitutionality of many of the powers seized by Congress in order to establish and finance that welfare state.

A more respectable objection to the idea of a normative as opposed to merely descriptive Law of Nature insists that it is impossible validly to deduce a normative conclusion from a purely descriptive premise. That, as a point of logic, is absolutely correct. But for Locke, and consequently for the Founding Fathers of the Republic, this Law of Nature was the system that would be or would have been prescribed by rational human beings in a State of Nature. And, just as no individuals in such a state could have any right to prescribe an item for inclusion in such a system unless they simultaneously accepted a reciprocal obligation themselves to obey that prescription, so no individual can reasonably claim a right to a liberty, or indeed to anything else, unless they are prepared simultaneously to accept an obligation to respect the corresponding rights of everyone else.[35]

The prescriptive laws of nature and the natural rights of man seem, at least by Locke himself, to have been conceived as arising from the essential nature of objects supposed to have been Divinely created rather than from *ad hoc* Divine endowments upon those objects. My academically justifying reason for suggesting this is that, in the second paragraph just quoted, Locke insists that the rights arising from the Law of Nature "should be equal one amongst another without Subordination or Subjection *unless* the Lord and Master of them all, should by any manifest, Declaration of His Will set one above another and confer on him...an undoubted Right to Dominion and all Sovereignty" (emphasis supplied). And that, of course, is precisely what Locke believes that he has in the *First Treatise* shown that God has *not* done.

But I myself have a less detachedly academic reason for wanting to show that the validity of the rights claims made in the Declaration of Independence is not logically dependent on a belief in the Divine creation of human beings. The reason is that that is a belief I myself am unable to share and is, for better or for worse, even in the United States, becoming progressively less universal. And I do not want respect for these natural rights to decline with any decline in belief in the Divine creation of the members of our species.

Three points need to be made about the claim in the Declaration "that all Men are created equal" before we return to Locke. The first, which will be universally acceptable today but certainly would not have been in 1776, is that the word "Men" should in future be construed as referring to all human beings of either sex; or, as the PC police insist, of either gender. The second is that we should construe the word "equal" as referring to our equality as creatures all possessing the essential and peculiar characteristics of human beings: above all the characteristic of being members of a most peculiar set who can and therefore cannot but make choices between the various alternative and often very different possibilities of action or inaction which are from time to time open to us as individuals. It is because some of these alternative possible choices could be made of our own free will and others only under various forms of coercion or constraint that freedom matters so much. The third point is a negative one, which did not need to be made in 1776 but, most emphatically, does need to be made today. It is that the Declaration does not assert either that all normal human beings are equally talented or even that the average ability across all racially or socially defined sets is the same.[36]

In the chapter from which the first two paragraphs have just been quoted Locke goes on to insist that although the State of Nature is "a *State of Liberty*, yet it is *not a State of License… The State of Nature* has a Law of Nature to govern it, which obliges every one: And Reason, which is that Law, teaches all Mankind, who will but consult it, that being all equal and independent, no one ought to harm another in his Life, Health, Liberty or Possessions."

Human beings, however, being human, there are bound to be transgressors. There has, therefore, even in the State of Nature, to be some provision for dealing with them. So, Locke goes on, "And that all men may be restrained from invading others' Rights, and from doing hurt to one another…the *Execution* of the Law of Nature is in that State, put into every Mans hands, whereby everyone has a right to punish the transgressors of that Law to such a Degree, as may hinder its Violation."

What next? Locke gives his answer in Chapter IX, "Of the Lands of Political Society and Government." It was that:

> If Man in the State of Nature be so free, as has been said…why will he part with his Freedom? To which 'tis obvious to Answer, that in the state of Nature he hath such a

right, yet the Enjoyment of it is very uncertain, and constantly exposed to the Invasion of others. This makes him willing...to joyn in Society with others who are already united, or have a mind to unite for the Mutual *Preservation* of their Lives, Liberties and Estates, which I call by the general Name, *Property*.

Locke therefore concluded that, "The great and *chief end* therefore, of Mens uniting into Commonwealths, and putting themselves under Government is *the Preservation of their Property*." The crucial Lockean conception of property is more comprehensive than the common contemporary notion. But thus, to preserve the people's property—in this understanding of the word "property" the "great and *chief end*...of Mens uniting into commonwealths, and putting themselves under Government..."—was to provide, as did the Founding Fathers of the American Republic, for an extremely limited form of government. It was this concern that led to the introduction of the first five Amendments to the Constitution, all restricting the powers of Congress, and the last of them ending "nor shall private property be taken for public use without just compensation."

When in peacetime during the nineteenth century any member of Congress suggested that taxes and money be voted for any charitable purpose, another member would surely ask what clause in the Constitution gave Congress the power to do this, and there came no answer. It should therefore not have been surprising that, when the Supreme Court was first asked to rule on the constitutionality of the major welfare measures of Roosevelt's first term, its ruling was negative.

Anyone who wonders how it is that a Constitution that was originally intended to provide for only a very limited government has come now to be interpreted in such a way as to provide for one that seems almost unlimited must take account, among many other things, of the enormous influence of John Rawls' *A Theory of Justice* upon the intellectuals in the thirty years since it was first published. This is a work that, I was recently told, is widely used in teaching about justice in those law schools from which America's future Supreme Court judges are most likely to come.

Notes

1. Cambridge, MA, Harvard University Press, 1971 and Oxford, Clarendon, 1972.
2. 1972, Issue 3.
3. *Atlantic* magazine for July 1953, p. 27. For what classical liberalism was, see, for instance, Conway 1995.
4. F. A. Hayek 1976, p. 31.

5. This work was traditionally subtitled "Concerning Justice," and has since been regarded as the first published treatise on that subject.
6. On this bizarre performance, Richard Hare, Regius Professor Moral Philosophy in the University of Oxford commented, in the second part of what must have been the longest of all the critical notices, that "Rawls…wishes to 'leave questions of meaning and definition aside and to get on with the task of developing a substantive theory of justice.' There is in fact a vast hole in his 600-page book which should be occupied by a thorough account of the meanings of these words, which is the only thing that can establish the logical rules that govern moral argument. If we do not have such an account, we shall never be able to distinguish between what we have to avoid saying if we are not to contradict ourselves or commit other *logical* errors, and what we have to avoid saying if we are to agree with Rawls and his coterie" (*The Philosophical Quarterly* 1973, p. 147). So much for what was elsewhere described as "the most substantial and interesting contribution to moral philosophy since the war."
7. *The Republic* 331E.
8. *Social Justice: Strategies for National Renewa*l (London: Vintage, 1994).
9. Ibid., p. ix.
10. Ibid., p. ix.
11. Ibid., p. 1.
12. Frankena, W., "The Concept of Social Justice," in R. B Brandt (ed.) 1956, p. 16.
13. Hayek, 1944, p. xi.
14. See note 7, chapter 5.
15. Rawls, 1971, p. 258.
16. Ibid., p. 62 (emphasis added).
17. Ibid., p. 137.
18. Ibid., p. 15 (emphasis added).
19. Ibid., p. 74.
20. Ibid., p. 74. For a reference to some discussion of this idea, see note 22, below.
21. Ibid., p. 150.
22. Ibid., p. 100. This conclusion must surely have been one of the most powerful stimuli to what Sowell, 1999 characterizes as "The Quest for Cosmic Justice." Who, by the way, could these individuals be to whom Nature is assumed to have allocated genes? For a critique of this misguiding picture of the human condition see Flew 1981, chapter IV.
23. Rawls, 1971, p. 60.
24. Ibid., p. 141.
25. Ibid., p. 150-1. By far the best account of the reasons why this principle appeared so obvious to Rawls and to so many of his contemporaries was provided by Robert Nisbet's "The Pursuit of Equality." This first appeared in *The Public Interest*, No. 35, Spring 1974, pp. 103-128.
26. Weale, 1978, p. 32.
27. Russell, B. A. W., 1919, p. 17.
28. Berlin, Isaiah, "Equality," in the *Proceedings of the Aristotelian Society*, Vol. LVI, LVI (1955-6), p. 305.
29. Stephen, James Fitzjames, 1873, p. 191 and compare Flew, 1981, chapter III.
30. Nozick, 1974, pp. 198-9.
31. Rawls, 1971, p. 15.
32. Rawls, 1971, pp. 15 and 179 (comma and emphasis added). This third assumption constitutes not only an unlovely dog in the manger commitment but also a commitment manifestly incompatible with the initial insistence upon "the priority of liberty."

I confess, not very shamefacedly, that had I discovered that my principles required such a commitment I should have taken that as a pressing reason for reviewing those principles.

33. In an article reprinted in Flew (ed.) 1951, pp. 11-36.
34. We happen to be brothers-in-law.
35. A pupil once asked Confucius whether his rule of conduct might be epitomized in a single word. "The Master replied, 'Is not "reciprocity" the word?' Do not do to others which you would not like yourself" (*Analects* XV, 23).
36. Anyone who actually wants to know the truth about this matter, and about how it has been and how it still is being denied and suppressed, should refer to such works as Rushton 1995, Snyderman and Rothman 1990, Pearson, Roger 1991, and Taylor, Jared 1999.

9

Moral Education in Secular State Schools

Mere justice is, upon most occasions, but a negative virtue, and only hinders us from hurting our neighbour. The man who barely abstains from violating either the person, or the estate, or the reputation, of his neighbours, has surely very little positive merit. He fulfils, however, all the rules of what is peculiarly called justice, and does everything which his equals can with propriety force him to do, or which they can punish him for not doing. We may often fulfil all the rules of justice by sitting still and doing nothing.
—*Adam Smith,* The Theory of the Moral Sentiments *(II, 1)*

Traditionally throughout the whole Western world the main moral teacher has been the family, usually reinforced by the church. Their work has sometimes been supplemented and sometimes undermined by such institutions of the wider society as the schools and the welfare and criminal justice systems. But in the UK there have, during the last forty or so years been both with regard to families and in the welfare and criminal justice systems, been developments that make both the need for and the difficulty of effective moral education in the schools greater than ever before. And there is in fact overwhelming evidence of a very substantial increase in the numbers of criminal offenses in England and Wales.

In the year ending March 2001, 5.2 million offenses in England and Wales were recorded by the police. This was about fifty-one times the rate in 1920 (when the population was only 37 million compared with 53 million today). It was about thirty-five times the rate in 1930 (147,000 crimes) and about eleven times the rate in 1950, when 461,000 crimes were recorded by the police and the population was 44 million. Crime did not pass the million mark until 1964, and it climbed steadily until it reached a peak of nearly 5.6 million in 1992. It currently seems to have reached a plateau of about eleven times the rate in the early 1950s. These criminal offenses were, almost without exception, such as most of us could scarcely fail to admit to have been also immoral.

Why Schools have become so Important

For fully two decades after the conclusion of World War II the position of the traditional family in the UK remained much the same as it had been in previous centuries. That is to say that almost all children were produced and raised by their biological parents, who had been married by, at the latest, the time of the birth of their first child, and who remained married until death did them part. But today, although the majority of men and women do marry and stay married to the same partners for the rest of their lives, and although the majority of children are still being raised by their biological parents, these majorities have become much less overwhelming, and are apparently still continuing to diminish, and hence may eventually disappear.

A spattering of statistics indicates the extent to which the institution of the traditional family has, in the UK, weakened during the last thirty or forty peacetime years. Between 1971 and 1991, the number of lone-parent households more than doubled (from 570,000 to 1,300,000). Up till 1984, nearly three-quarters of the increase was attributable to the rise in divorced and separated mothers. But lone parenthood is increasingly the result of a huge and historically unprecedented increase in single motherhood, and almost all these single mothers and their children are being supported by the state welfare system. Whereas the proportion of births to unmarried women had never at any time in the two centuries and more since reliable national statistics first became available exceeded 7.5 percent, and had in most years been considerably lower, it stood at the time of writing at 30 percent. This is the highest figure for any of the present fifteen member states of the European Union. Apparently the statistics for the remaining countries of the geographers' Europe are not available.

What makes all this crucially relevant to us here is the extremely robust social scientific finding that the children of parents who do not follow traditional norms (i.e. undertaking a personal, active, long-term responsibility for the upbringing of the children of whom they are the biological parents) are thereby disadvantaged in many major ways. The abundant available evidence[1] shows that such children tend to die earlier, to suffer more illness, to do less well at school, to suffer more unemployment, to be more delinquent, and, finally, to go on to repeat the cycle of unstable parenting from which they themselves have suffered.

Perhaps the most important way in which moral education is provided by the general society outside its homes and schools is through the criminal justice system, and in particular in and through the treatment of the youngest and presumably most impressionable offenders. For more than three decades, with the best of intentions but with what would appear to have been the most deplorable results, successive steps have been taken to make the English criminal justice system less punitive towards youngsters.

The effect has been that young offenders can be confident that not much is going to happen to them for any offense short of a major felony—and maybe not even then. This is particularly true of offenders in their early teens. Only 10 percent of all youths aged under fourteen who were picked up by the police in 1994 for an indictable offense were even found guilty of anything, let alone given any considerable punishment. The rest were merely cautioned—let go, with no further action whatsoever, after a few minutes' lecture from a policeman. Compare this with 1954: among those under age fourteen who were picked up 77 percent were, having been indicted, found guilty.[2]

The significance of this abandonment of punishment is perhaps most strongly suggested by the following statistic. In 1954, a year during which England experienced only one-eleventh the number of indictable offenses that it experienced in 1994, more than six times as many youths under the age of fourteen were found guilty of indictable offenses: 19,865 in 1954 compared with 3,200 in 1994.[3] No doubt many other causes played some part in producing this huge increase in juvenile crime. For few if any interesting social phenomena are mono-causal. But only a truly heroic apologist for those anti-punishment policies would dare to deny that they had made a very substantial contribution.

Why our State Systems must be Secular

From the end of World War II until the passing of the 1988 Education Reform Act (ERA), the British state-maintained school system and the U.S. public school system, though of course in many ways very different, were nevertheless more like each other than either was like the system of any state on the European mainland. Under neither of these systems would it today be practically possible to promote an ethic based on a religion, although the reasons for this are different in the two cases.

It is also here necessary to discount the existence in the UK of a substantial minority of originally religious foundations that are now largely funded by tax money. There should be no objection to the teaching of, as opposed to about, a religion or a religion-based ethic in such schools, just so long as a right of withdrawal from the relevant periods of instruction is granted for dissident parents.

Despite the fact that there is an abundance of evidence suggesting that there is in the U.S. substantially more religious belief and religious practice than in any European countries other than Poland and Ireland, we find that the Supreme Court has for many years been insisting that the First Amendment to the Constitution is to be construed as requiring a "wall of separation" between church and state. That amendment reads:

> Congress shall make no law respecting an establishment of religion, or prohibiting the free exercise thereof; or abridging the freedom of speech, or of the press, or the right of the people peaceably to assemble, and to petition the Government for a redress of grievances.

The situation with regard to moral and religious education in the UK is more complicated. It is sufficient here to start by saying that in 1944, the year of the passage of the Education Act which was to shape the UK state-maintained school system until the passage of the Education Reform Act (ERA) in 1988, there were two established churches: the Church of England in England, and the Kirk of Scotland in Scotland. The work of getting representatives of these two established churches plus representatives of several other denominations to produce an agreed national syllabus for Religious Education (RE) occupied an inordinately disproportionate amount of the working time of the cabinet minister responsible for the production of the Bill which became this Act.[4]

At that time no official distinction seems to have been made between religious and moral education. It was apparently assumed that, after the passage of that 1944 Act, and with the consequent introduction of a period of RE and the provision for acts of worship in regular school assemblies, both had been provided for simultaneously and sufficiently. Certainly no notice was taken of warnings of the unfortunate practical implications of that equation in a period that was likely to and in fact did see a massive decline in vigorous religious belief and practice.

Already in 1982 the Church of England was, as we saw in chapter 4 above, showing signs of being, in more than one sense, in secular decline. For it then appeared to have a greater commitment to the promotion of social justice than to the promotion of Christianity as traditionally understood. Earlier, in his contributions to a collection of essays entitled *The Myth of God Incarnate*,[5] the then-Regius Professor of Divinity at the University of Oxford, who was also chairman of the Church of England's Doctrine Commission, had argued that the conception of an incarnate God would appear to be irremediably self-contradictory. Later, in the 1980s, David Jenkins, bishop of Durham, confirmed the suspicions raised earlier by *Faith in the City*.[6] For he not only denounced the policies of Prime Minister Thatcher as "wicked," but himself dismissed claims that Jesus rose from the dead as "a conjuring trick with bones."[7]

It is surely significant that, throughout the 1980s, the archbishop of Canterbury was Robert Runcie. For he had during the 1960s been principal of Cuddesdon, a theological college that produced many bishops, and in which David Jenkins was at that time a lecturer. Apparently it was in those days a hotbed of what would previously have been accounted heresy.[8]

In view of these radical changes in what might be comprehensively described as the religious belief situation since 1944, no one ought to have been surprised to discover that those who drafted the Bill that was to become the 1988 Education Act made no provision for RE. They must have realized that such provision would need somehow to take account not only of the decline in the belief in and the practice of the Christian religion, but also of the very substantial growth in the numbers of Hindus, Sikhs, and, above all, Muslims. What eventually resulted after a great deal of conflict and confusion was a law about RE in state-maintained schools that is being widely disobeyed, with tacit ministerial support for the disobedient.

A Propagandizing False Start

The 1988 Education Reform Act called for the introduction of a compulsory ten-subject National Curriculum, which has to be followed in all state-maintained schools. That Act eventually contained a clause stating that that National Curriculum should promote the "spiritual, moral, cultural, mental and physical development of the pupils at the school and of society." When in 1996 the School Curriculum and Assessment Authority (SCAA), a body established under the ERA, eventually realized that something had at last to be done to implement the clause requiring the National Curriculum to promote—inter alia[9]—"the moral...development of pupils at the school and of society," the results were, expectedly, shambolic. It summoned a National Forum on Values in Education and the Community. This was directed to attempt to produce consensus. The ostensible success of this attempt was guaranteed in part by the careful choice of members and in part by the peculiarly restrictive methods imposed on its operation. This Forum eventually produced its findings in the form of a document entitled *Consultation on values in education and the community.*

The most remarkable thing about the whole exercise was how far removed it was from elementary moral education as traditionally understood. That was a matter of teaching individuals the difference between right and wrong in the simplest, most primitive, and most fundamental contexts, and the success of such pedagogic performances in schools required not the mere communication of information but inducing the pupils actually and habitually to obey the dos and to eschew the don'ts, primarily and immediately in the contexts of school life.

But this *Consultation* document started by listing—in the section "The Values" and under the subheading "Society"—the values that "we as a society" supposedly cherish. It then went on to list what were seen as corresponding principles of action: "On the basis of these values, we as a society should..." Many of those principles are in consequence such as simply could not be moral rules for, and followed by, every individual individually. Instead they are principles directed at society in general. In effect this amounted to saying "the state," and calling on citizens to support all manner of tax-funded welfare services.

Consider for instance, the commands: "to provide opportunities for all," and to "support people who cannot sustain a dignified lifestyle by themselves." Those aware that "social" justice is different from, and incompatible with, old-fashioned, without prefix or suffix justice are bound to feel even more uneasy when they notice that in this *Consultation* document the word "justice" is found only under the sub-heading "Society."

In its concluding columns, headed "Principles for Action," many of the crucially relevant distinctions are not made. In it we are, for instance, under the subheading "Relationships," required as one of our "principles for action" to "respect the beliefs...of others." But this requirement fails to distinguish between respecting someone's right to hold and to express a belief and respecting the content of that belief. One could respect all beliefs regardless of their content only at the cost of abandoning or never acquiring any concern about the truth of propositions, the validity of arguments, or anything much else. But by its failure to make and to insist upon this absolutely fundamental and crucial distinction, this *Consultation* document does its bit to sustain the currently fashionable standardless relativism as applied to questions both of truth and of morality. Such comprehensively generalized relativism, which would better be described as subjectivism, and that requires that we all refuse to be judgmental about or otherwise to stigmatize any particular type of behavior, is altogether incompatible with the maintenance of any generally accepted standards of morality.

It is scarcely likely that anyone seeking consensus about some fundamentals of right and wrong would have sought it by establishing a Forum on Values in Education and the Community. Instead they would have attempted to excogitate fundamental principles that might be universally agreed upon—what I once heard an influential Oxford philosopher describe as the "plain moral facts."

But the primary concern of SCAA was very different. For the practices it wanted to justify included exercises in what is known as "values clarification."[10] This seems to be an intellectual descendant of John Dewey's theory of citizenship and it has certainly been, at least until very recently, much more prevalent in the USA than in the UK. It is important to recognize that these exercises are radically incompatible with any education in any morality of which the principles are equally mandatory on all who are confronted with what are in the relevant respects the same circumstances. These exercises are, that is to say, totally incompatible with teaching any morality at all.

This comes out very clearly from statements in one of the most widely recommended textbooks: "An increasing number of students are no longer willing to tolerate a curriculum that does not acknowledge their needs, interests and concerns. Schools, as well as homes, must offer young people a way to develop a set of values upon which they can act and base their lives. How do young people acquire a set of values? Are we to tell them what to value and how to live, over and over again, in the hope that they will listen? No. *None of us can be certain that our values are right for other people*" (emphasis added).[11]

Values clarification thus categorically eschews what any program of moral education necessarily attempts. For it is, at least theoretically and professedly, indifferent to the values eventually adopted by those subjected to courses of values clarification. It is sufficient that their individual and personal values should be *full* values and, as such, chosen freely, chosen from among alternatives, chosen after due reflection, prized and cherished, publicly affirmed, acted upon, and part of a pattern that is a repeated action.

Is there any one of these criteria that was not fully, indeed most abundantly, satisfied by the values of Adolph Hitler in his promotion and implementation of the Holocaust? *The Sun*, Britain's favorite tabloid, dismissed the whole preposterous business of "values clarification" in a characteristically robust editorial entitled "No Choice." That concluded: "Morality is about sticking to a strict code of right and wrong—not choosing your own values. *We'll be letting kids choose whether they murder old ladies next.*"[12]

The Essentials of Social Morality

The obvious candidates for inclusion in even the most minimal syllabus of moral education are the principles of what, in view of the enormous popularity of that misleadingly mistitled book of Rawls, we have now to qualify as old-fashioned, without prefix or suffix justice. In the year 1739, in Book III of *A Treatise of Human Nature*, David Hume published what was surely the first totally secular and this-worldly account of the origin of what he and in his day everyone else took to be, at least in a legal context, the necessarily connected ideas of justice and property. (It is here relevant to add that as soon as it was published Hume gave a copy of this work to his young friend Adam Smith.)

The first step in Hume's treatment "Of justice and injustice" is for us the most significant. For he started by asserting that justice is one of those virtues "that produce pleasure and approbation by means of an artifice or contrivance which arises from the circumstances and necessity of mankind."[13] Such virtues are in the *Treatise* uneasily characterized as artificial. But in his later *Enquiry concerning the Principles of Morals* he substituted the here truly appropriate word "social." This substitution was right. For justice as here understood is the virtue that is essential to any tolerable social living.

That is why in *The Theory of the Moral Sentiments*, the work from which the motto of the present chapter is drawn, Adam Smith began his own classic discussion of justice by distinguishing it as a virtue "of which the observance is not left to the freedom of our own wills" but "which may be extorted by force..."; adding that the violation of justice is injury—it does real and positive hurt to some particular persons. His conclusion here is that: "The man who is barely innocent, who only observed the laws of justice with regard to others, and merely abstains from hurting his neighbours, can merit only that his neighbours in their turn shall respect his innocence."

This conclusion is for us most significant. For it tacitly appeals to what is surely the fundamental principle of the most rudimentary moral education, the principle of the negative Golden Rule: "Do not do to others what you would not willingly permit them to do to you." It is to that principle that parents and other moral teachers are appealing when they ask an aggressive child: "How would you like it if I did the same to you?" It was not for nothing that, when a pupil asked him whether his rule of conduct could be epitomized in a single word, Confucius (551-479 B.C.) replied, "Is not 'reciprocity' the word?"[14] This response is peculiarly appropriate to our present secularizing purposes. For Classical Chinese apparently contained no ideograph for the concept of God. Thus, when the first Jesuit missionaries arrived at the Court of the Emperor of China and started to translate parts of the Bible into Chinese, the best they could do was to render the Latin Deus into the Chinese T'ien, the ideograph usually rendered into English as "Heaven."[15] The ethics of Confucius therefore were, and could not but have been, totally secular.

It was in what was later to become also Smith's understanding of the socially essential nature of justice that Hume, in a section of the *Treatise* entitled "Of the origin of justice and property," had gone on to urge that, while the conception of a state of nature "is, no doubt, to be regarded as an idle fiction," nevertheless it "deserves our attention, because nothing can more evidently show the origins of those virtues, which are the subjects of our present enquiry."[16] The attention that Hume granted to this supposedly idle fiction—to which, as we saw earlier in the section entitled "Justice as Fairness or Justice as Justice?" in chapter 8, Locke was able to give so much profitable employment—enabled him to conclude that, "without justice, society must immediately dissolve, and every one must fall into that savage and solitary condition, which is infinitely worse than the worst situation that can possibly be suppos'd in society."[17] So what Hume was doing in this section was producing a speculative but nevertheless plausible account of the natural evolution as opposed to the planned and directed introduction of certain fundamental moral ideas and practices.

This sketch for a secular and evolutionary account of the moral norms essential for any tolerable social life may now be profitably compared with that given in Wallace Matson's most illuminating article on "The Expiration of Morality."[18] This article develops the notion of the "low morality" that would have been essential to what are believed to have been the original human hunter-gatherer societies. That morality is continuous with the morality of sub-human gregarious animals, and is basically the same for all human groups, being a specification of how "normal" people must habitually behave if a community is to be viable. Precisely how those requirements are to be realized will of course vary with the size, complexity, and capabilities of the particular groups.

Here Matson makes a suggestive comment: "The low morality…is concerned with the *right* (thing to do) and not with The Good, some shining ideal condition to the realisation of which individual or social effort must be directed… Low morality is not concerned with ultimate aims, as long as they are not incompatible with doing the right thing; and this leaves much leeway. As far as low morality goes, it is all right to pursue wealth or learning, or political power, or pleasure, as long as the means employed are above board."[19] Values clarifiers could surely make their activities at least consistent with, if not a form of, moral education if only they were prepared to insist that to be acceptable any values so clarified must presuppose an unequivocal commitment to the principles of low morality. For, as Matson insists, "the necessary conditions for a viable society are everywhere the same. *There is no alternative to low morality*."[20]

Two further points made here by Matson are relevant to our present inquiry. Both employ his distinction between low and high morality and both concern religion. He argues first, that whereas "*low* morality is constant and transcends tribal boundaries, it is only the common core of actual comprehensive moralities, which [these] exhibit much variety. The variable element I...call *high* morality."[21] This variable element was originally a product of religion, and, "since the *modi operandi* of the gods, as well as their names, natures, sexes and other attributes, are all products of mere imagination, the beliefs and rituals about them will vary more or less at random from tribe to tribe. That is to say, high beliefs and the practices based on them, "—the *high* morality—unlike low beliefs and practices, will not be uniform; what is believed and done on this side of the mountain and the other side will be 'diverse.'"[22]

The second relevant point to be made in the light of Matson's distinction between low and high morality is that it is itself invaluable equipment for moral educators who have to deal with, and, hopefully, to dispose of, the moral relativism that today seems to be endemic in the schools of the Western world. For, as Matson himself insists, it is reports of the differences between the high moralities of different tribes that "lead to the belief that morals are 'relative.' In a way they are; but only in a way. What is really plural is religion (and the *high* morality derived from it), not the rules as to how it is necessary to behave if a society—any society—is to be viable (*low* morality)."[23]

Is this Syllabus Sufficient?

There are two questions here. The first is, are there any further essentials that must be included in any syllabus for secular moral education? And the second is, is it possible and desirable to include anything more than essentials in what it is hoped could become an agreed-upon syllabus of moral education?

Given our realization that any morality to be taught in the state schools of either the UK or the USA cannot but, for better or for worse, be secular; and now given also both Hume's account of how such a naturalistic system might have evolved and Matson's very similar account of what he calls "low morality," we can now return to repeat Locke's account of the heart of the matter:

> The *State of Nature* has a Law of Nature to govern it, which obliges every one: And Reason, which is that Law, teaches all Mankind, who will but consult it, that being all equal and independent, no-one ought to harm another in his Life, Health, Liberty or Possessions.

Certainly the Law of Nature is here seen as a system that prescribes the principles of justice. But while there can be no doubt but that a general rule to speak the truth has to be included in any syllabus for the teaching of a low morality for today, since social cooperation with people who cannot be relied on normally to speak the truth is extremely difficult if not altogether impossible, it is not so clear that this is a rule of justice. Certainly any system of justice has to criminalize perjury. But perjury is always intentionally saying what is false in certain peculiar circumstances. The offense of perjury thus resembles offending against the Ninth Commandment, "Thou shall not bear false witness against thy neighbour," in that it forbids only one sort of lying. Since no one would deny that the enforcement of legitimate contracts is a proper function of even the most limited governments, we may perhaps take it for granted that it is justice that demands that (at least morally legitimate) promises must be kept. The alternative approach would be to argue that to lie to people is to insult them, that to insult someone is to hurt or otherwise harm them, and hence to conclude that the forbidding of lying would be, like the forbidding of the violation of any of the (other) principles of justice, a forbidding of the doing of harm to other people.

Unquestionably the essentials of a low morality are principles forbidding the doing of any actual harm to other people. But there should surely be a place in any syllabus for moral education for some attempt to inspire at least some of those being morally educated with ideals of doing some kind of positive good. I do not know how this is to be done. For few of the "celebrities" nowadays so strenuously publicized by the media seem ever to have felt any obligation "to set a good example." So the best I can do—at the cost of provoking a chorus of sneers against my "Victorian values" from all properly left-thinking people—is to assert that what is needed, but perhaps can never be provided, is an enormously popular book of biographies that would do for the twenty-first century what Samuel Smiles 1866 did for the nineteenth and after.

In view of what was said in the section about "The Rise of Single Motherhood and the Decline of the Family" in chapter 3, it would clearly be wrong to conclude the present work without at least raising the question of whether any further prescriptions are needed in order to produce an adequate low morality for the UK and the USA today.

When it came to questions about sexual activity and the production and the raising of children, Hume—and indeed until some time in the twentieth century just about everyone else in all the countries of Christendom—took the traditional Christian family and its traditional norms absolutely for granted. The Fifth and the Seventh Commandments are susceptible of some sort of a purely secular justification. For although unbelievers will understandably be unmoved by the incentive promised in the command to "Honor thy father and thy mother: that thy days may be long upon the land which the Lord thy God giveth thee," we all surely ought to acknowledge some obligation to help our parents if and when they become too old to help themselves. And the authority for the proscription of adultery lies in the terms of the marriage contract of which the act of adultery would necessarily be a breach. If and in so far as marriage involves a contract to live together, forsaking all others, "till death do us part," the expression "no fault divorce" must be strictly self-contradictory, and a substantial breach of marriage vows becomes an offense morally equivalent to that of perjury.

For us here the problem is fornication, which it may be remembered, is not one of the sorts of action forbidden by any of the Ten Commandments. Providing that it is completely consensual, and does not result in pregnancy and the production of children, I can see no purely secular and this-worldly objection. But that proviso is crucially important. Accumulating discoveries about the effects of a fatherless upbringing surely determine duties not to act in ways likely to produce children who will be raised without the cooperation of a father. The burden of duty thus imposed would fall in a satisfactorily non-sexist way equally upon men and women. The duty would be not to engage in sexual intercourse unless both partners are willing and able, and if their actions should in fact result in the birth of a child, would fully to cooperate in the upbringing of that child.

Towards the end of his discussion on "Of Morals" in the *Treatise*, Hume opines "that reflections on the tendencies of actions have by far the greatest influence, and determine all the great lines of our duty."[24] The tendency of actions of the kind forbidden by the present proposed moral rule is to produce children who will not be raised as well as they could and should be. These actions also tend to produce single mothers whose support, with that of their offspring, constitutes a heavy and continuing burden upon the unfortunate taxpayers.[25]

But be warned, if we accept this consequentialist moral argument for a duty not to act in ways likely to produce children who will be raised without the cooperation of a father, we may find ourselves having, however reluctantly, to admit that Vice President Dan Quayle was right the first time—and wrong only in his later retraction. For he had objected, it may be remembered, to the heroine of a prime time TV sitcom "mocking the importance of fathers" and to her calling her decision to have a baby while unmarried "just another lifestyle choice." Such "moralist stigmatising provoked outrage," with editorial writers and talk show hosts criticizing him for "a bludgeoning attack on unmarried mothers."[26]

Notes

1. For this see the sections entitled "The Rise of Single Motherhood and the Decline of the Family" and "What is to be Done?" of chapter 3, above and the notes thereto.
2. For the sources of these and further relevant statistics, and for a demolition of claims that these figures have been misinterpreted to produce a baseless "moral panic" see Dennis and Erdos 1992 and compare Dennis 1993.
3. For the sources of these statistics and a discussion of their significance, see Murray 1977.
4. This has been known since it was offered as the all too plausible excuse for the failure to do more to meet the long recognized national need for more and better technical education.
5. Hick, John, (ed.), 1977; compare Wiles 1999.
6. O'Brien (Chairman), 1985.
7. I have myself argued more than once both in public debates and in published articles that the evidence is altogether insufficient to establish this miraculous conclusion. But I have never expressed my disbelief so offensively, and never would.
8. See Dennis, Norman, 2001, pp. 48-9. This book can be strongly recommended to anyone wishing to know more about the history of the involvement of the Church of England in school, as opposed to university, education.
9. Anyone interested in the problem of measuring spiritual development when the word "spiritual" is emphatically not to be construed as synonymous with the word "religious" can be referred to Flew and Naylor 1996.
10. For its impact in the UK, see Seaton 1995.
11. Simon, Sidney, Howe, Leland, and Kirschenbaum, Howard, *Clarifying Values through Subject Matter: Applications for the Classroom* (Minneapolis: Hart, 1973), p. 31; emphasis supplied.
12. October 20, 1994 (emphasis original).
13. III(ii), 1, p. 477.
14. *Analects*, XV, 23.
15. It is said that when news of this heretically impersonal rendering reached Rome the missionaries were rebuked. Certainly "T'ien" still does not mean "God." If it did, the militantly atheist regime would not tolerate the theological implications of the name "T'ienanmen Square!"

16. III(ii), 2, p. 494.
17. III(ii), 2, p. 497.
18. In Paul, E. F., Miller, E. D., and Paul, J. (eds.), *Cultural Pluralism and Moral Knowledge* (Cambridge: Cambridge University Press, 1994), pp. 159-178.
19. Ibid., p. 165 (emphasis original).
20. Ibid., p. 166 (emphasis original).
21. Ibid., p. 166 (emphasis original).
22. Ibid., pp. 168-9 (emphasis original).
23. Ibid., p. 169 (emphasis original).
24. III(iii) 1, p. 590.
25. In the UK, taxpayers presently contribute to this undeserving cause roughly eight billion pounds a year, a sum very similar to that paid out annually by our unfunded national pension system.
26. See *The Sunday Times* (London) for May 29, 1992, "Quayle shoots from the lip as Bush flounders." One has to wonder whether the journalists who write in this way would be equally hostile to moralizing, stigmatizing, or "bludgeoning attacks" if those attacked or stigmatized were alleged racists or alleged homophobes, and, if not, why not?

Bibliography

Anderson, Digby (ed.) (1), *The Ignorance of Social Intervention* (London: Croom Helm 1980).

Anderson, Digby (ed.) (2), *The Kindness that Kills: The Churches' Simplistic Response to Complex Social Issues* (London: SPCK, 1984).

Anderson, Digby (ed.) (3), *Full Circle? Bringing Up Children in the Post-Permissive Society* (London: Social Affairs Unit, 1988).

Anderson, Digby (ed.) (4), *The Loss of Virtue: Moral Confusion and Social Disorder in Britain and America* (New York and London: National Review and Social Affairs Unit, 1992).

Anderson, Digby (ed.) (5), *This Will Hurt: The Restoration of Virtue and Civic Order* (New York and London: National Review and Social Affairs Unit, 1995).

Anderson, Digby (ed.) (6), *Gentility Recalled: 'Mere' Manners and the Making of Social Order* (London and Grand Rapids, MI: Social Affairs Unit and Acton Institute for the Study of Religion and Liberty, 1996).

Anderson, Digby (ed.) (7), *Full Circle? Bringing Up Children in the Post-Permissive Society* (London: Social Affairs Unit, 1998).

Anderson, Digby and Dawson, G. (eds.), *Family Portraits* (London: Social Affairs Unit, 1986).

Anderson, Digby, Lait, J., and Marsland, D., *Breaking the Spell of the Welfare State* (London: Social Affairs Unit, 1981).

Anderson, Digby and Mullen, P. (eds.), *Faking It: The Sentimentalism of Modern Society* (London: Social Affairs Unit, 1998).

Aristotle (384-322 BC), *Politics*, translated by Ernest Barker (Oxford: Clarendon, 1948).

Aristotle (384-322 BC), *Nicomachean Ethics*, translated by H. Rackman (Cambridge, MA and London: Harvard U.P. and Heinemann, 1977).

Austin, J. L., *Sense and Sensibilia* (Oxford: Clarendon, 1962).

Bainton, R. H., *Here I Stand: A Life of Martin Luther* [1950] (New York: New American Library, 1954).

Bork, Robert, *Slouching Towards Gomorrah: Modern Liberalism and American Decline* (New York: Harper Collins, 1996).

Borrie, Gordon (ed.), *Social Justice: Strategies for National Renewal* (London: Vintage, 1994).

Borzellieri, Frank, *The Unspoken Truth: Race, Culture and Other Taboos* (Oakton, VA: New Century, 1999).

Bramah, Ernest, *The Wallet of Kai Lung* (London: Jonathan Cape, 1900 with innumerable reprintings thereafter).

Brandt, R. B. (ed.), *Social Justice* (Englewood Cliffs, NJ: Prentice Hall, 1965)
Brewer, Colin and Lait, J., *Can Social Work Survive?* (London: Temple Smith, 1980).
Burke, Edmund, *Reflections on the Revolution in France* [1790], edited and introduced by Conor Cruise O'Brien (London: Penguin, 1968).
Burn, John, Marks L., Pilkington, P., and Thompson, P., *Faith in Education: A Response to the Dearing Report on Church Schools in the Third Millennium* (London: Civitas, 2001).
Carroll, Lewis, *The Collected Works of Lewis Carroll*, with an Introduction by Alexander Woolcott (London: Nonesuch, 1939).
Chall, J. S. *The Academic Achievement Challenge* (New York, Guilford Press, 2000).
Chew, Jennifer, *Spelling Standards: How to Correct the Decline* (London: Centre for Policy Studies, 1996).
Chubb, J. E. and Moe, T. M., *Politics, Markets and America's Schools* (Washington, DC: Brookings Institution, 1990).
Colebatch, Hal, *Blair's Britain* (London: Claridge, 1999).
Confucius (559-471 BC), *The Analects*, in Vol. I of *The Chinese Classics*, translated and annotated by James Legge (Hong Kong and London: "at the author's" and Trubner, 1861).
Conway, David, (1), *Free-Market Feminism* (London: IEA Health and Welfare Unit, 1998).
Conway, David (2), *Classical Liberalism: The Unvanquished Ideal* (New York and London: St. Martin's and Macmillan, 1995).
Cox, Caroline and Marks, J. (1), *Sixth Forms in ILEA Comprehensives: A Cruel Confidence Trick* (London: National Council for Educational Standards, 1980).
Cox, Caroline and Marks, J. (eds.) (2), *The Right to Learn* (London: Centre for Policy Studies, 1982).
Darwin, Charles, *The Origin of Species* [1859] (London: Penguin, 1968).
David, Miriam E. (ed.), *The Fragmenting Family: Does it Matter?* (London: IEA Health and Welfare Unit, 1998).
Davies, Christie, *Permissive Britain* (London: Pitman, 1975).
Davies, Jon (ed.), *The Family: Is it Just Another Lifestyle Choice?* (London: IEA Health and Welfare Unit, 1993).
Deacon, Alan (ed.), *Ending Dependency: Lessons from Welfare Reform in the USA* (London: Civitas, 2001).
Dennis, Norman, (1), *Rising Crime and the Dismembered Family* (London: Institute of Economic Affairs, 1993).
Dennis, Norman (2), *The Invention of Permanent Poverty* (London: IEA Health and Welfare Unit, 1997).
Dennis, Norman (3), *The Uncertain Trumpet: A History of Church of England School Education to AD 2001* (London: Civitas, 2001).
Dennis, Norman and Erdos, G., *Families with Fatherhood* (London: IEA Health and Welfare Unit, 1992). Third Edition incorporating fresh and more recent materials, 2000.

Dennis, Norman, Erdos, G., and Al-Shahi, A., *Racist Murder and Pressure Group Politics: The Macpherson Report and the Police* (London: Civitas, 2000).
Dennis, Norman and Halsey, A. H., *English Ethical Socialism* (Oxford: Oxford U.P., 1998).
D'Souza, Dinesh, *Illiberal Education: The Politics of Race and Sex on Campus* (New York: The Free Press, 1991).
Duncan, Alan and Hobson, Dominic, *Saturn's Children: How the State Devours Liberty, Prosperity and Virtue* (London: Sinclair-Stevenson, 1995).
Eberstadt, Nick, *The Poverty of Communism* (New Brunswick, NJ and London: Transaction Publishers, 1988).
Efron, Edith, *The Apocalyptics: How Environmental Politics Controls What We Know about Cancer* (New York: Simon and Schuster, 1984).
Ellis, Frank, *The Macpherson Report: 'Anti-racist' Hysteria and the Sovietization of the United Kingdom* (London: Right Now, 2001).
Epstein, Richard A., *Forbidden Grounds: The Case Against Employment Discrimination Laws* (Cambridge, MA: Harvard U.P., 1992).
Flew, Antony (1), *An Introduction to Western Philosophy: Ideas and Argument from Plato to Popper* [1971] (London: Thames and Hudson, 1989).
Flew, Antony (2), *Sociology, Equality and Education: Philosophical Essays in Defence of a Variety of Differences* (London: Macmillan, 1976).
Flew, Antony (3), *A Rational Animal: Philosophical Essays on the Nature of Man* (Oxford: Clarendon, 1978).
Flew, Antony (4), *The Politics of Procrustes: Contradictions of Enforced Equality* (London and Amherst, NY: Temple Smith and Prometheus, 1981).
Flew, Antony (5), *Education, Race and Revolution* (London: Centre for Policy Studies, 1984).
Flew, Antony (6), *Darwinian Evolution* [1984] (New Brunswick, NJ and London: Transaction Publishers, 1997).
Flew, Antony (7), *Thinking About Social Thinking* [1985] (Amherst, NY: Prometheus, 1995).
Flew, Antony (8), *Merely Mortal? Could You Survive Your Own Death?* [1987] (Amherst, NY: Prometheus, 2000).
Flew, Antony (9), *Power to the Parents: Reversing Educational Decline* (London: Sherwood, 1987).
Flew, Antony (10), *Equality in Liberty and Justice* [1989] (New Brunswick, NJ and London: Transaction Publishers, 2001).
Flew, Antony (11), *A Future for Anti-Racism?* (London: Social Affairs Unit, 1992).
Flew, Antony (12), *Shephard's Warning: Putting Education Back on Course* (London: Adam Smith Institute, 1994).
Flew, Antony and Macintyre, Alasdair (eds.), *New Essays in Philosophical Theology* (London, SCM Press, 1955).
Flew, Antony and Naylor, Fred, *Spiritual Development and All That Jazz* (York: Campaign for Real Education, 1996).
Freeman, Derek (1), *Margaret Mead and Samoa: The Making and Unmaking of an Anthropological Myth* (Cambridge, MA, and London: Harvard U.P., 1983).

Freeman, Derek (2), *The Fateful Hoaxing of Margaret Mead: A Historical Analysis of Her Samoan Research* (Boulder, CO: Westview, 1999).
Giddens, Anthony, *The Third Way: The Renewal of Social Democracy* (London: Polity, 1998).
Green, David G. (1), *Benefit Dependency: How Welfare Undermines Independence* (London: IEA Health and Welfare Unit, 1988).
Green, David G. (2), *Reinventing Civil Society: The Rediscovery of Welfare Without Politics* (London: IEA Health and Welfare Unit, 1993).
Green, David G. (3), *Community without Politics: A Market Approach to Welfare Reform* (London: IEA Health and Welfare Unit, 1996).
Green, David G. (4), *An End to Welfare Rights: The Rediscovery of Independence* (London: IEA Health and Welfare Unit, 1999).
Green, David G. (ed.), *Underclass: The Crisis Deepens* (London: IEA Health and Welfare Unit, 1994).
Green, David G. (ed.), *Institutional Racism and the Police: Fact or Fiction?* (London: Civitas, 2000).
Hayek, F.A. (1), *The Constitution of Liberty* (Chicago and London: Chicago U.P. and Routledge and Kegan Paul, 1960).
Hayek, F.A. (2), *The Road to Serfdom* [1944] (London and Henley, Routledge and Kegan Paul, Second Edition 1976).
Hayek, F.A. (3), *Rules and Order*, Vol. I of his trilogy on *Law, Legislation and Liberty* (London: Routledge and Kegan Paul, 1973).
Hayek, F.A. (4), *The Mirage of Social Justice*, Vol. II of his trilogy on *Law, Legislation and Liberty* (London and Henley: Routledge and Kegan Paul, 1976).
Hayek, F.A. (5), *The Political Order of Free People*, Vol. III of his trilogy on *Law, Legislation and Liberty* (London: Routledge and Kegan Paul, 1979).
Hernstein, R. J., *IQ in the Meritocracy* (Boston: Atlantic–Little Brown, 1973).
Hernstein, R. J. and Murray, Charles, *The Bell Curve: Intelligence and Class Structure in American Life* (New York: The Free Press, 1944).
Hick, John (ed.), *The Myth of God Incarnate* (London: SCM Press: 1977).
Himmelfarb, Gertrude (1), *The Idea of Poverty: England in the Early Industrial Age* (London and Boston MA, Faber and Faber, 1984).
Himmelfarb, Gertrude (2), *The De-moralization of Society: From Victorian Virtues to Modern Values* (London: IEA Health and Welfare Unit, 1995).
Himmelfarb, Gertrude (3), *One Nation, Two Cultures* (New York: Vintage, 2001).
Hitchens, Peter, *The Abolition of Britain* (London: Quartet, 1999).
Hobhouse, L. T., *Elements of Social Justice* (London: Allen and Unwin, 1922).
Honeyford, Ray (1), *Integration or Disintegration: Towards a Non-Racist Society* (London and Lexington, KY: Claridge, 1988).
Honeyford, Ray (2), *The Commission for Racial Equality: British Bureaucracy and the Multiethnic Society* (New Brunswick, NJ and London: Transaction Publishers, 1998).
Horowitz, David, *Hating Whitey, and Other Progressive Causes* (Dallas, TX: Spence Publishing, 1999).
Hoskyns, John, *Just in Time: Inside the Thatcher Revolution* (London: Autumn, 2000).

Hoover, K. and Plant, Raymond, *Conservative Capitalism in Britain and the United States: A Critical Appraisal* (London: Routledge, 1989).
Housman, A. E. *Juvenalis Saturae* [1905] (Cambridge: Cambridge U.P., Revised Edition, 1931).
Hume, David (1), *A Treatise of Human Nature* [1739], edited by L.A. Selby-Bigge, revised by P.H. Nidditch (Oxford: Clarendon, 1979).
Hume, David (2), *Enquiries Concerning the Human Understanding and Concerning the Principles of Morals* [1748 and 1752], edited by L.A. Selby-Bigge, revised by P. H. Nidditch (Oxford: Clarendon, 1979).
Huxley Julian (1), *Essays of a Biologist* [1923] (Harmondsworth: Penguin, 1939).
Huxley, Julian (2), *Evolution in Action* (London: Chatto and Windus, 1953).
Jensen, A. R., *Genetics and Education* (Edinburgh: Constable, 1972).
Jouvenel, Bertrand de, *The Ethics of Redistribution* [1951] (Indianapolis, IN: Liberty Fund, 1990).
King, Martin Luther Jr., *Testament of Hope: The Essential Writings of Martin Luther King Jr.* (San Francisco: Harper and Row, 1986).
Kirby, Jill, *Broken Hearts: Family Decline and the Consequences for Society* (London: Centre for Policy Studies, 2002).
Kitcher, Philip, *Vaulting Ambition, Sociobiology and the Quest for Human Nature* (Cambridge, MA: Massachusetts Institute of Technology, 1985).
Kors, A. C. and Silvergate, H. A., *The Shadow University: The Betrayal of Liberty on America's Campuses* (New York: The Free Press, 1998).
Kurtz, Paul and Madigan, Timothy (eds.), *Challenges to the Enlightenment* (Amherst, NY: Prometheus, 1994).
Lammers, S. E. and Verhey, A., *On Moral Medicine: Theological Perspectives in Medical Ethics* (Grand Rapids, MI: Erdman, 1987).
Le Fanu, James, *A Phantom Carnage: The Myth that Low Income Kills* (London: Social Affairs Unit, 1993).
Lefever, Ernest W., *Amsterdam to Nairobi: The World Council of Churches and the Third World* (Washington DC: [Georgetown] Ethics and Public Policy Center, 1979).
Letwin, Oliver, *Beyond the Causes of Crime* (London: Centre for Policy Studies, 2002).
Lewis, W. A., *The Principles of Economic Planning* (London: The Fabian Society, 1949).
Lister, Ruth (ed.), *Charles Murray and the Underclass: The Developing Debate* (London: IEA Health and Welfare Unit, 1996).
Locke, John (1), *Two Treatises of Government* [1690], edited by Peter Laslett (Cambridge: C.U.P., 1960).
Locke, John (2), *An Essay Concerning Human Understanding* [1690], edited by Peter H. Nidditch (Oxford: Clarendon, 1979).
Lynn, Jonathan and Jay, Antony, *The Complete Yes Minister* (New York: Harper and Row, 1988).
Lynn, Richard (1), *Educational Achievement in Japan: Lessons for the West* (London: Macmillan and Social Affairs Unit, 1988).

Lynn, Richard (2), *The Secret of the Miracle Economy: Different National Attitudes to Competition and Money* (London: Social Affairs Unit, 1991).
Macintosh, J. J. and Meynell, H. A. (eds.), *Faith, Scepticism and Personal Identity: A Festschrift for Terence Penelhum* (Calgary: University of Calgary Press, 1994).
Macpherson, Sir William, *The Stephen Lawrence Enquiry: Report of an Inquiry by Sir William Macpherson of Cluny* (London: Stationery Office, 2000).
Malinowski, Bronislaw, *Sex and Repression in Savage Society* (London: Routledge and Kegan Paul, 1927).
Malthus, T. R., *An Essay on the Principle of Population* [1798], edited with an Introduction by Antony Flew (Harmondsworth,: Penguin, 1970).
Mandeville, Bernard de, *The Fable of the Bees* [1729], edited by P. Harth (Harmondsworth: Penguin, 1970).
Marks, John (1), *Standards of Arithmetic: How to Correct the Decline* (London: Centre for Policy Studies, 1996).
Marks, John (2), *The Betrayed Generations: Standards in British Schools 1950-2000* (London: Centre for Policy Studies, 2000).
Marks, John (3), *Grammar Schools in the Twenty-First Century* (Oldbury: National Grammar Schools Association, 2001).
Marks, John (4), *Standards and Spending: Dispelling the Spending Orthodoxy* (London: Centre for Policy Studies, 2002).
Marsland, David, (1), *Seeds of Bankruptcy: Sociological Bias Against Business and Freedom* (London: Claridge, 1988).
Marsland, David (2), *Welfare or Welfare State: Contradictions and Dilemmas in Social Policy* (New York: St. Martins, 1996).
Martin, David, *Tongues of Fire: The Explosion of Protestantism in Latin America* (Cambridge, MA and Oxford, Blackwell, 1989).
Marx, Karl, *The Eighteenth Brumaire of Louis Bonaparte* [1852] (London, Progress, 1934).
Marx, Karl and Engels, Friedrich, *The Communist Manifesto* [1848], translated by S. Moore (Harmondsworth: Penguin Books, 1968).
Matthews, Kent and Benjamin, Dan, *US and UK Unemployment between the Wars: A Doleful Story* (London: Institute of Economic Affairs, 1992).
Miller, David, *Social Justice* (Oxford: Clarendon, 1976).
Minogue, Kenneth, *The Silencing of Society: The True Cost of the Lust for News* (London: Social Affairs Unit, 1997).
Mitchell, William C., *Government As It Is* (London: Institute of Economic Affairs, 1988).
Mitchell, William C. and Simmons, Randy T., *Beyond Politics: Markets, Welfare and the Failure of Bureaucracy*, (Boulder, CO: Westview Press, 1994).
Montagu, Ashley, *Sociobiology Examined* (Oxford: Oxford University Press, 1980).
Morgan, Patricia (1), *Farewell to the Family: Public Policy and Family Breakdown in Britain and the USA* (London: IEA Health and Welfare Unit, 1950). The new updated and expanded edition of 1999 does not include the statements of the Law Commission quoted in the text above.

Morgan, Patricia (2), *Adoption and the Care of Children. The British and American Experience* (London: IEA Health and Welfare Unit, 1988).

Morgan, Patricia (3), *Who Needs Parents? The Effects of Childcare and Early Education on Children in Britain and the USA* (London: IEA Health and Welfare Unit, 1996).

Morgan, Patricia (4), *Marriage-Lite: The Rise of Cohabitation and its Consequences* (London: Institute for the Study of Civil Society, 2000).

Morris, Desmond, *The Human Zoo* (London: Cape, 1970).

Murray, Charles (1), *Losing Ground, American Social Policy, 1950-1980* (New York: Basic Books, 1984).

Murray, Charles (2), *In Pursuit of Happiness and Good Government* (New York and London: Simon and Schuster, 1988).

Murray, Charles (3), *The Emerging British Underclass* (London: IEA Health and Welfare Unit, 1990).

Murray, Charles (4), *Underclass: The Crisis Deepens* (London: IEA Health and Welfare Unit, 1994).

Murray, Charles (5), *Does Prison Work?* (London: Institute of Economic Affairs, 1997).

Norman, Edward, *Christianity and the World Order* (Oxford: O.U.P., 1979).

Novak, Michael, *Will it Liberate? Questions about Liberation Theology* (Mahwah, NJ: Paulist Press, 1986).

O'Keeffe, Dennis, *Political Correctness and Public Finance* (London: Institute of Economic Affairs, 1999).

O'Keeffe, Dennis (ed.), *The Wayward Curriculum* (London: Social Affairs Unit, 1986).

Olasky, M., *The Tragedy of American Compassion* (Washington DC: Regnery Gateway, 1992).

Palmer, Frank, *Anti-Racism: An Assault on Education and Value* (London: Sherwood, 1986).

Pappas, Theodore, *Plagiarism and the Culture War: The Writing of Martin Luther King Jr. and Other Prominent Americans* (Tampa, FL: Halberg, 1998).

Parker, Hermione, *The Moral Hazard of Social Benefits: A Study of the Impact of Social Benefits and Income Tax on Incentives to Work* (London: Institute of Economic Affairs, 1982).

Pearson, Roger, *Race, Intelligence and Bias in Academe* (Washington, DC: Scott Townsend, 1991).

Phillips, Melanie (1), *All Must Have Prizes* (London: Little, Brown and Company [UK], 1996).

Phillips, Melanie (2), *America's Social Revolution* (London: Civitas, 2001).

Philpot, Terry (ed.), *Political Correctness and Social Work* (London: IEA Health and Welfare Unit, 1999).

Plato, *The Republic,* with English translation by Paul Shorey (London and Cambridge, MA: William Heinemann and Harvard U.P., 1935).

Price, R. H., Ketter, R. F., Bader, B. C., and Monahan, J. (eds.), *Prevention in Mental Health: Policy and Practice* (Beverley Hills, CA and London: Sage, 1980).

Pryke, Richard, *A Critique of Low-Income Statistics: Alternative Estimates and Policy Implications* (London: Institute of Economic Affairs, 1995).
Quest, Caroline (ed.), *Equal Opportunities: A Feminist Fallacy* (London: IEA Health and Welfare Unit, 1992).
Quest, Caroline (ed.), *Liberating Women...from Modern Feminism* (London: IEA Health and Welfare Unit, 1994).
Radnitsky, G. and Bouillon, H. (eds.), *Values and the Social Order*, Vol. 2 (Aldershot: Avebury, 1995).
Rawls, John, *A Theory of Justice* (Cambridge, MA and Oxford: Harvard U.P., 1971 and Clarendon, 1972).
Richardson, Ken and Spears, David (eds.), *Race, Culture and Intelligence* (Harmondsworth: Penguin, 1972).
Richman, Sheldon, *Separating School and State* (Fairfax, VA: The Future of Freedom Foundation, 1994).
Robbins, Lionel, *The Nature and Significance of Economic Science* (London: Macmillan, 1932).
Roberts, Paul Craig and La Follette, Karen, *Meltdown: Inside the Soviet Economy* (Washington, DC: The Cato Institute, 1990).
Rowen, Henry and Wolf, Charles (eds.), *The Impoverished Superpower: Perestroika and The Soviet Military Burden* (San Francisco: Institute for Contemporary Studies, 1990).
Runyon, Damon, *Runyon on Broadway* (London: Constable, 1950).
Rupp, E. G., Marlow, A. N., Waterson, P. S., and Drewery, B. (eds. and translators), *Luther and Erasmus: Freewill and Salvation* (Philadelphia, PA: Westminster, 1969).
Rushton, J. Phillippe, *Race, Evolution and Behaviour* (New Brunswick, NJ and London: Transaction Publishers, 1995).
Ruskin, John, *Unto this Last* (London: G. Allen, 1899).
Russell, B.A.W. (1), *An Introduction to Mathematical Philosophy* (London: Allen and Unwin, 1919).
Russell, B.A.W. (2), *Freedom and Organisation 1814-1914* (London: Allen and Unwin, 1934).
Sacks, Jonathan, *Wealth and Poverty: A Jewish Analysis* (London: Social Affairs Unit, 1985).
Sandberg, Nils-Eric, *What Went Wrong in Sweden?* (Stockholm: Timbro, 1997).
Sartre, Jean-Paul, *Being and Nothingness* (London: Methuen, 1957).
Schaler, Jeffrey A. and Schaler, Magda. E. (eds.), *Smoking: Who Has the Right?* (Amherst, NY: Prometheus, 1998).
Schoek, H., E*nvy: A Theory of Social Behaviour*, translated by M. Glenny and B. Ross (London: Secker and Warburg, 1969).
Seaton, Nick, *New Gods for Schools: Self, Society, Relationship and the Environment* (York: Campaign for Real Education, 1995).
Seldon, Arthur, *Charge* (London: Temple Smith, 1977).
Seldon, Arthur (ed.), *Reprivatizing Welfare: After the Last Century* (London: Institute of Economic Affairs, 1996).
Sheppard, David, *Bias to the Poor* (London: Hodder and Stoughton, 1983).

Sherrington, Charles, *Man on His Nature* (Cambridge: Cambridge University Press, 1940).
Sirico, R., *A Moral Basis for Liberty* (London: Institute of Economic Affairs, 1994).
Skinner, B.F., *Beyond Freedom and Dignity* (New York and London: Knopf, 1971 and Cape, 1972).
Smiles, Samuel, *Self-Help with Illustrations of Conduct and Perseverance* [1859] (London: IEA Health and Welfare Unit, 1996).
Smith, Adam (1), *The Theory of the Moral Sentiments* [1759] (Oxford: Clarendon, 1976).
Smith, Adam (2), *An Inquiry into the Nature and Causes of the Wealth of Nations* [1776] (Indianapolis, IN: Liberty Press, 1981).
Smith, Alwyn and Jacobsen, B. (eds.), *The Nation's Health: A Strategy for the 1990s* (London: King Edward's Hospital Fund for London, 1988).
Smith, Bernard, *The Fraudulent Gospel: Politics and the World Council of Churches* [1977] (Richmond, Surrey: Foreign Affairs Publishing, Third Enlarged Edition, 1991).
Snyderman, Mark and Rothman, Stanley, *The IQ Controversy: The Media and Public Policy* (New Brunswick, NJ and London: Transaction Publishers, 1990).
Sowell, Thomas (1), *Knowledge and Decisions* (New York: Basic Books, 1980).
Sowell Thomas (2), *Ethnic America* (New York: Basic Books, 1981).
Sowell, Thomas (3), *The Economics and Politics of Race* (New York: William Morrow, 1983).
Sowell, Thomas (4), *Civil Rights, Rhetoric or Reality* (New York: William Morrow, 1984).
Sowell, Thomas (5), *Education: Assumptions versus History* (Stanford, CA: Hoover Institution, 1986).
Sowell, Thomas (6), *Preferential Policies: An International Perspective* (New York: William Morrow, 1990).
Sowell, Thomas (7), *Inside American Education: The Decline, The Deception, The Dogmas* (New York: The Free Press, 1993).
Sowell, Thomas (8), *Race and Culture: A World View* (New York: Basic Books, 1994).
Sowell, Thomas (9), *The Vision of the Anointed: Self-Congratulation as Basis for Social Policy* (New York: Basic Books, 1995).
Sowell, Thomas (10), *Migrations and Cultures: A World View* (New York: Basic Books, 1996).
Sowell, Thomas (11), *Conquests and Cultures: An International History* (New York: Basic Books, 1998).
Sowell, Thomas (12), *The Quest for Cosmic Justice* (New York: The Free Press, 1999).
Sowell, Thomas (13), *A Personal Odyssey* (New York: The Free Press, 2000).
Stephen, James Fitzjames, *Liberty, Equality and Fraternity* (London: Smith and Elder, 1873).
Tawney, R. H. (1), *The Acquisitive Society* (London: G. Bell, 1921).

Tawney, R. H. (2), *Equality* (New York: G. Bell, Third Revised Edition, 1938).
Tingle, Rachel, *Another Gospel?* (London: Christian Studies Centre, 1998).
Tocqueville, Alexis de, *Memoir on Pauperism*, translated by Seymour Drescher (London: IEA Health and Welfare Unit, 1997).
Tooley, James (1), *Disestablishing the School: Debunking Justifications for State Intervention in Education* (London: Institute of Economic Affairs, 1996).
Tooley, James (2), *Reclaiming Education* (London and New York: Cassell, 2000).
Tooley, James (3), *The Global Education Industry* [1999] (London: Institute of Economic Affairs, 2001).
Tullock, Gordon (1), *The Vote Motive* (London: Institute of Economic Affairs, 1976).
Tullock, Gordon (2), *The Economics of Wealth and Poverty* (New York: New York U.P., 1986).
Tullock, Gordon (3), *The Economics of Non-Human Societies* (Tucson, AZ: Pallas Press, 1994).
Tullock, Gordon, Seldon, Arthur, and Brady, Gordon L., *Government: Whose Obedient Servant?* (London: Institute of Economic Affairs, 2000).
Turner, Martin and Burkard, Tom, *Reading Fever: Why Phonics Must Come First* (London: Centre for Policy Studies, 1996).
Weale, David, *Equality and Social Policy* (London: Routledge and Kegan Paul, 1978).
West, Edwin G. (1), *Education and the State: A Study in Political Economy* [1965] (Indianapolis: Liberty Press, 1994).
West, Edwin G. (2), *Education and the Industrial Revolution* (London: Batsford, 1975).
Wharton, Michael, *Peter Simple's Century* (London: Claridge, 1999).
Whelan, Robert (1), *The Corrosion of Charity: From Moral Renewal to Contract Culture* (London: IEA Health and Welfare Unit, 1996).
Whelan, Robert (2), *Involuntary Action: How Voluntary is the 'Voluntary' Sector?* (London: IEA Health and Welfare Unit, 1999).
Whelan, Robert (ed.), *Teaching Right and Wrong: Have the Churches Failed?* (London: IEA Health and Welfare Unit, 1994).
Whelan, Robert (ed.), *Just a Piece of Paper? Divorce Reform and the Undermining of Marriage* (London: IEA Health and Welfare Unit, 1995).
White, Margaret (1), *Children and Contraception—Time to Change?* Edited by Joanna Bogle (London: Order of the Christian Unity Press, 1994).
White, Margaret (2), *The Safe Sex Hoax*, edited by Joanna Bogle (London Order of the Christian Unity Press, 1999).
Wiles, Maurice, *Reason to Believe* (London, SCM Press, 1999).
Wilkinson, Richard G., *Unhealthy Societies: The Afflictions of Inequality* (London and New York, Routledge, 1996).
Williams, Walter E. (1), *The State against Blacks* (New York: McGraw-Hill, 1982).
Williams, Walter E. (2), *All it Takes is Guts: A Minority View* (Washington, DC: Regnery Gateway 1987).

Williams, Walter E. (3), *Do the Right Thing: The People's Economist Speaks* (Stanford, CA: Hoover Institution Press, 1995).
Williams, Walter E. (4), *More Liberty Means Less Government: Our Founders Knew This Well* (Stanford, CA: Hoover Institution Press, 1999).
Wilson, E. O. (1), *The Insect Societies* (Cambridge, MA: Harvard University Press, 1971).
Wilson, E. O. (2), *Sociobiology: The New Synthesis* (Cambridge, MA: Harvard University Press, 1975).
Wilson, E. O. (3), *On Human Nature* (Cambridge, MA: Harvard University Press, 1978).
Wilson, James Q., *Thinking About Crime* [1975] (New York: Vintage 1977).
Wolfe, B. D., *Marxism: One Hundred Years in the Life of a Doctrine* (London: Chapman and Hall, 1967).

Name Index